Healing Hashimoto's

A Savvy Patient's Guide

Dr. Alan Christianson

Copyright © 2013 by Alan Christianson, NMD

Printed in the United States of America

First Printing, 2013

ISBN 978-1481205351

Integrative Health Care Publishing
9200 East Raintree #100
Scottsdale, AZ 85260

www.integrativehealthcare.com

Introduction

Welcome to Healing Hashimoto's, a Savvy Patients Guide!

A lot has happened in the thyroid world since Hy Bender and I wrote The Complete Idiot's Guide to Thyroid Disease.

Since the rate of new cases of thyroid disease is only increasing, many still need introductory material as found in The Complete Idiot's Guide to Thyroid Disease. This still serves as my favorite overview of hypothyroidism, hyperthyoridism and thyroid cancer.

The most common type of thyroid disease is hypothyroidism and in the modern world, the most common cause of hypothyroidism is Hashimoto's Thyroiditis. Medical treatment guidelines focus only on thyroid hormone replacement. Mind you this is with precious little finesse in dosing and very few medication options.

The new trend is that many people with thyroid disease have become much more savvy. Social media is a large factor in this. Gena Lee Nolin, former Baywatch star, created an amazing movement with her Facebook page, Thyroid Sexy. People have shared their experiences in ways that has really escalated the population's level of understanding and therefore also the depth of information they need.

In addition, authors such as Mary Shomon, Dr. Mark Starr, Dr. Datis Kharrazian and Janie Bowthorpe have also promoted a deeper understanding of the condition and its optimal treatment.

Hashimoto's Thyroiditis is an complex interaction of genes, environmental toxins, nutrients, the immune function and other hormones. Consequently, many patients need correction in a unique combination of these areas to really feel their best.

The purpose of this book is to serve the savvy, educated patient who is questing to regain their optimal health. For those who have done the basic steps and still are not at your best, this is for you.

The content I'm sharing is a distillation of many sources. My initial sources of information were medical school with an early interest in thyroid disease and then post medical training and education from sources including:

- American Academy of Clinical Endocrinology

- American Thyroid Association

- Broda Barnes Foundation

- Denis Wilson, MD

Since 1996, my main area of focus in private practice has been thyroid disease and natural endocrinology. I've logged over 50,000 patient visits related to these conditions in this timeframe. People come in not because I'm the doctor on their HMO plan, not because I'm nearby and not because I'm easy to get into. They come in because they have heard I can help and that I really care.

The cool thing I get to witness on a daily basis is people getting better. For me the ultimate high is to play a part in this process.

What sparked a young med student's obsession with thyroid disease? Jamie's story and my story may explain this.

Jamie's story

During one of my first clinical shifts, I had the opportunity to work with 'Jamie'. She was 15 and had debilitating fibromyalgia. Her pain and fatigue were so bad, she had to withdraw from school a few months before I saw her. She had seen many doctors, none found any underlying reasons for her fibromyalgia and none had found treatments that gave her more benefits than side effects.

As a naive student, I thought about her symptoms: fatigue, muscle pain, edema, weight gain, depression, sleep disturbances. To me it sounded just as much like thyroid disease as fibromyalgia. When I looked in her chart, she did have basic thyroid labs done and they were normal. I asked one of the doctors about this. He told me that prior doctors thought this and tried to give Jamie thyroid treatment. All it did was give her anxiety and palpitations while worsening her insomnia. "Besides, her labs were normal", he reminded me.

Too stubborn to let it go, I talked to Jamie and her mom about this. It turned out her mom had similar issues in her mid twenties, many of which improved when she was diagnosed with and treated for thyroid disease. Jamie's mother said the prior doctor did try thyroid treatment with Jamie but she was started at a 2 grain dose of Armour Thyroid. They wondered if this was just too much initially.

My supervising doctor was willing to do further testing per my request. After doing more detailed blood tests and an ultrasound, it was apparent that Jamie did have Hashimoto's Thyroiditis even though her gland was not abnormal by basic tests.

By starting her on gentle treatment she was able to improve. Over the first 3 months she lost 15 pounds and was able to go back to school. Jamie still visits me about once a year. She lives across the country with her husband and children. She was able to finish high school and college and get her life back.

My story

I resonated with Jamie because I was also a sickly adolescent. At 12 years of age I was at my all time low. I was grossly obese and had zero physical coordination. This was the result of epilepsy early in life. As a child my brain was lousy at some things but exceptional at others. I read my family's Wold Book Encyclopedia set cover to cover before kindergarten.

After an especially humiliating gym class, I used what I had and went to the library. Over a few weeks I read dozens of books on medicine, fitness, nutrition and health. I made a plan and I worked my butt off, quite literally. In two years I was lean and fit. Having never played organized sports I made it to the starting team in football and was the fastest runner of all ages during training sessions.

It was like I was trapped under ice and was able to find hole to get out. Jamie made me realize that people with thyroid disease were trapped under ice but didn't always have a rescue hole. Both conventional and alternative medicine did not always have adequate options. I saw that they both had parts of the puzzle but really had not put it together. I felt compelled to do so and did.

This book represents my findings from this journey in an accessible format. It is intentionally written in a conversational and practical format. Imagine that we were seated next to each other on a LA to New York flight and you told me you had Hashimotos. This book would be that conversation.

As you read this remember that an ounce of practice equals a ton of theory. If you read something here you've read before, before dismissing it ask yourself, are you living it? If you are not at your optimal health and you find steps that you may not be following completely, please commit to acting on them completely for two months before dismissing them. If you see possible triggers or culprits, before thinking they don't apply to you, get tested. If you have been tested already, were you treated and did the results improve? If not don't give up. If you were tested and the results were normal, did you have the most accurate tests read by someone experienced?

Hopefully you can see the thought process it takes to get better. You need to find the highest priority thing that can be slowing you down and stay on it until it is completely resolved. Once this is done, address the next factor. As you'll learn, this can be food intolerances, allergies, chronic infections, environmental toxins, adrenal issues or just being on the wrong dose of thyroid.

Never give up on yourself, you can get better!

Alan Christianson, NMD

Scottsdale, AZ - 2013

Reviews

"In helping people overcome weight loss resistance, I have seen how hard thyroid disease can be to correct hypothyroidism. Whenever someone has really been stuck because of their thyroid, I've connected them with Dr. Alan Christianson. He has consistently been able to help them get their thyroid levels right. It has been nothing short of amazing to see how big of an impact this has on their weight and overall well being. "

JJ Virgin, author of NY Times bestseller <u>The Virgin Diet: Drop 7 Foods, Lose 7 Pounds, Just 7 Days</u>.

"Dr. Alan Christianson has done a great job synthesizing conventional and alternative approaches to thyroid disease. I've enjoyed collaborating with him on these topics and recommend his work to anyone seeking clarity on Hashimoto's Disease."

Alan Gaby, Author, <u>Nutritional Medicine textbook</u>. Expert in nutritional therapy

"Dr. Alan Christianson offers a credible voice in discussing thyroid disorders. His detailed understanding and practical clinical experience provides guidance that you can trust in helping you improve your health."

Michael T. Murray, N.D., co-author of <u>The Encyclopedia of Natural Medicine</u>

"Dr. Alan Christianson is my favorite thyroid guru. He loves the science as much as I do, and has a rare gift for translating complex information into delightfully clear language.

"Over the years he has helped countless people with thyroid disease get their health back on track. He walks the talk, and lives and breathes robust health on a daily basis.

"His work is engaging, compelling, and conversational. You can really understand the concepts and take simple effective steps that will help you revive your vitality!"

Sara Gottfried, MD, Author of <u>The Hormone Cure</u>

Contents

Introduction   *i*

Chapter 1 Thyroid Overview   1

Chapter 2 Ins and Outs of Hashimotos'   17

Chapter 3 Optimize Your Dose   33

Chapter 4 Losing Weight   57

Chapter 5 Best and Worst Foods   75

Chapter 6 Hashis' Happens, Here's Why   89

Chapter 7 Getting Your Thyroid Squeaky Clean   103

Chapter 8 Best and Worst Pills for Your Thyroid   113

Chapter 9 Healing Your Adrenals   129

Chapter 10 Healing your Nervous System   145

Closing   152

Chapter 1

Thyroid Overview

Chapter At a Glance

- Welcome

- Three aspects of Hashimoto's Disease - Immune function, thyroid hormone levels, thyroid gland structure.

- 'Hows' and 'Whys' of Thyroid function

- Role of Toxins

- Genetic susceptibility

- Salt and Iodine

Welcome to this series. This is about healing Hashimoto's for the well-informed patient. I want to thank all of you so much for your interest. When I put this audio series and book together, it was for the exact purpose of helping clarify many issues unique to those who have Hashimoto's Disease. Mostly, they have not been given much direct attention. This is true although their condition is the most common cause of hypothyroidism, one of the most common diseases in America having the biggest effect on the largest number of people. Those who have active Hashimoto's have needs beyond merely replacing the lacking hormones, and people are becoming more and more aware of that. They realize that just taking a replacement pill, especially like a T4-only medication, will not take care of all their symptoms and issues, as there are other parts of it to manage.

When I think about Hashimoto's I always think about the three primary areas. With Hashimoto's you have an alteration in hormone production, an immune disease, and structural problems with the thyroid. The three of these are all domains that overlap. They also require separate attention for your health to optimize and to prevent other complications like thyroid cancer. Therefore, I put the word out to people – "What are some of your biggest challenges? What are your biggest questions?" and I was surprised to see that most questions were more about things like mechanisms and what I call the "hows" and the "whys" of Hashimoto's – "How did this happen? Why did this happen? What is the thyroid? How does this all play out?" so I am extremely pleased and happy to address those questions with the other important ones about "How can you feel better and how can we reverse your symptoms, help get your weight back to where it should be, get your energy back up, help your hair become healthier again?"

Therefore, we are going to cover that. In addition, in this first portion I am going to cover more of the causes – more of the mechanisms – and if this is of your interest – splendid. Hang out with me, and we will have a real fun trip through the entire world of what the gland does, where it is, and what the history of it is too. If that does not interest you, please jump to the relevant disk or chapter and get right into what matters to you. You will not hurt my feelings. In fact, I probably will not even know.

So moving right ahead... The thyroid, its job is to make hormones that dictate how our cells form energy, obviously an important task. Our cells are like individual people. They are kind of like separate things. They have their own skin, and they have their own organs, and if they work right then we work right and if they do not we do not. Therefore, none of them produces energy or makes proteins unless the right amount of thyroid hormone causes them do this. Therefore, it is critical to every cell from head to toe and because of that, any symptom you could imagine could be related to the wrong amount of thyroid hormone. Some symptoms are more likely related than others are but almost any symptom is possible, and is a long list of ways how it can affect our health.

The gland itself is not that large. It is about sixty grams, roughly the weight of a deck of cards yet its functions are vital. In addition, it works primarily by taking up this mineral called iodine. The unique relationship between iodine and the thyroid gland does not exist with other minerals or other parts of the body. Most minerals you could think of – things like magnesium or iron or zinc – individually they have more than a hundred jobs they do in the body. Those jobs are carried out by several parts of your body including your liver or your intestinal tract or your muscles or your brain. Therefore, every mineral you can think of does many things in many different areas. Now iodine has exactly one job and exactly one location for that unique job. The only essential thing we know it does in the body is to help the thyroid form hormones and is only done inside the thyroid. Often, iodine is found in other parts of the body. We excrete a little in our sweat, we pass it out in our urine, and small amounts are in breast milk, otherwise it is not known to be vital to any other structures in the body.

Therefore, within the gland, iodine is absorbed and the amount of iodine that flows through our blood is insufficient to form our thyroid hormones. Therefore, what happens is that the thyroid concentrates iodine by a mechanism called the sodium-iodine transport or sodium-iodine symport. In addition, it concentrates iodine anywhere from thirty to one hundred-fold over the amount found in the bloodstream. Consequently, much higher levels of iodine occur inside the gland than outside.

Many wastes circulating in our bodies are chemically like iodine. They can also become trapped in this pump and brought up inside the gland, which is one of the reasons that the thyroid gland can get diseased. Therefore, it concentrates iodine and it has to convert iodine chemically into thyroid hormones. Thyroglobulin is a protein that helps this conversion happen. Within the gland, the iodine is added to tyrosine and they are paired to make a new molecule. So think about tyrosine as T, then iodine as a number and when you hear about T4 or T3, all they mean is how many iodine atoms you have paired on a tyrosine. The various hormones – T4, T3, and T2 – serve different purposes in the body but they are just iodine and tyrosine. Nothing more complex than that.

The process is the gland mostly makes T4 but it makes a little T3 and T2. But after the hormone is released then the rest of your body – your organs like your liver or your kidneys but also each individual cell – has the ability to convert this T4, into T3 and T2, the more active products. Therefore, T4 is easy for the gland to secrete, it is not active alone, and that allows many levels of control over your thyroid. Your tissues and your cells and your liver – all of them have ways of modulating and using your hormone in various fashions based on your needs. Because this hormone is so powerful and vital, there are many checks and balances.

We think about those that go on kind of below the thyroid after the hormone is secreted and those that go on above the thyroid and control how much hormone it secretes. So your liver, your kidneys, your cells but also your intestinal tract – mechanisms by which the amount of hormone is converted, how it is converted, how it is eliminated – can be adjusted and varied to reach your body's needs. Aside from your thyroid gland in your brain, the primary things that control it are the hypothalamus and the pituitary. The pituitary is a little thing about the size and shape of a pea that sits just above your sinuses with the means to register how much thyroid hormone is in your blood, and based on that it stimulates the gland. In addition, it makes a hormone called thyroid-stimulating hormone and it is controlled itself by the hypothalamus. The hypothalamus makes the thyroid hormone into a releasing hormone that makes the pituitary work.

So I think about it as a corporation and the hypothalamus is the CEO, the pituitary is the manager, then in this context, the thyroid is one of the workers. Other workers would include the ovaries, the testicles, and the adrenal glands but today we are concerned more about the thyroid. The pituitary and the hypothalamus – they are the overseers of the thyroid – dictate how much hormone it makes. The thyroid takes up iodine and tyrosine, makes hormone out of that and releases it, then the body has many levels of control that determine how that hormone gets used – a mechanism for the formation and secretion of hormone.

Now when we look at medical history it is fascinating. Thyroid disease was one of the first things that we figured out in medicine that we still carry a similar understanding of today, for example, a disease called "goiter" that still happens with thyroid disease. In the past – in history – in other parts of the world, it was a much more common issue. In fact, in America at the turn of the century some areas, as many as a third of children in schools would have some degree of goiter. In addition, goiter is an enlargement of the thyroid. It is a rather diffuse enlargement so it is not a distinct nodule or mass but it is more so an overall swelling of the gland. This can occur for several reasons. The most common one is just a lack of iodine. Therefore, when there is not enough iodine, the gland is not putting out adequate hormone and that causes the pituitary to secrete more TSH. Because not enough hormone is coming out, even after the TSH elevates, the gland merely increases in size, which is the best it can do to compensate, but it is not helpful. This enlargement can get quite pronounced, unsightly, uncomfortable, disfiguring, and dangerous. It can be a big deal.

As much as 2,500 years ago, the Chinese had worked out that if you gave someone who had a goiter burned seaweed or if you gave them glandular tissue – thyroid glandular tissue from an animal – that would reduce the swelling in their neck. That was one of the first connections between a nutrient or a hormone and a disease process ever made. The same understanding holds true today. We know that iodine, which can come from seaweed, can treat a goiter and prevent it or reverse it if it is there. In addition, even today for conditions like hypothyroidism, we give glandular thyroid and it is an effective strategy. So this has been known about for so, so long in medical history – one of the first findings that still remains solid.

We now talk about Hashimoto's – our focus of this will be Hashimoto's – the most common reason that the gland is slowing in America today. In the rest of the world, iodine deficiency is a more common culprit. Here in the states, we have adequate amounts of iodine – we will talk in detail about iodine – but we have more danger to face from excessive iodine than from deficiencies of iodine. Therefore, we will bear that in mind as we proceed.

However, the cycle that occurs is that our body can attack the gland by mistake. Doctor Hashimoto identified this at the turn of the last century – and it is not a coincidence it showed up there. They have high rates of thyroid disease and that has been tied to their high intake of iodine. The typical Japanese, based on recent data, consumes about 2,500 micrograms (2.5 milligrams) of iodine per day, whereas in the states we consume about 300 to 400 micrograms (0.3 milligrams) per day on average, so they consume a lot more.

Now we talked before about how the gland pumps iodine inside itself. Well that pump works so hard that whenever you get too much iodine it makes the thyroid shut itself off for a little while and if it did not it would make so much hormone that it could damage your heart and hurt you. It could be a dangerous thing. Therefore, this shutoff mechanism is critical to prevent excess hormone from pouring out of your thyroid and hurting you. However, when the shutoff mechanism turns off and the gland starts operating again, it does not always come back perfectly and because of that, iodine in higher intakes can trigger thyroid disease. The shutting off and resetting of the gland can damage it, which is why they have higher rates of thyroid disease in Japan and that includes hypo, hyper and thyroid cancers.

Therefore, Hashimoto's Disease is actually on the rise in the modern world. There has been data saying the rates have been increasing during the last several decades. This is becoming more common as other autoimmune diseases becoming more common. Because it is a function of the body attacking itself, we do consider it an autoimmune reaction. A large tie-in between waste in the environment and errors in the immune system involves the body attacking itself. Therefore, as our world becomes more polluted, as people spend more time living in a polluted world, and as we have older people who had pollution earlier in their life and toxins earlier in their life, we see higher rates of autoimmune disease including thyroid disease. In many ways, thyroid disease can show up at lower levels of exposure to toxins than other autoimmune disease can and the reason for that goes back to that iodine concentrating mechanism.

With iodine other wastes can get concentrated inside the thyroid and that causes them to reach levels much higher than they would be in the muscle tissue or in the liver. Therefore, because of that the thyroid is kind of like the canary in the coalmine of the body. You may have heard of that expression before. In the past, miners knew they had a risk of being exposed to toxic gases in the mines but they did not have good machines or mechanisms to help them measure that and know when their exposure was starting before someone would get sick. Therefore, the practice was to bring a canary and the birds would sing practically all the time. They were a little more sensitive to the gases in the mines than people were. Therefore, when the bird quit singing it was time to get the heck out. That meant the miners were becoming toxic. Thankfully, now they have more humane ways of measuring that, and that metaphor is true of our thyroid. It is a first indicator of a problem due to toxic exposure with our bodies, and these things are rising.

Three basic steps are involved in making it happen – susceptibility, the toxins, and then the trigger. Therefore, susceptibility means genetic susceptibility and this is why this disease is more common if a family member has it. If a sibling or a first-degree relative, such as a parent, has it, then the chances of it occurring are much higher, especially for women. The disease has about an 8:1 female-male ratio so men do get it – not as commonly. Many have speculated that the exposure of fetal tissue to the mother's immune system makes it more common. And women actually have different immune systems for that reason because they have the capacity of harboring essentially a foreign life and not attacking it – and because of that they get the unlucky burden of having higher rates of autoimmune disease in general and this is one of those.

The complete cluster, including genetic susceptibility, which can include variations in how well you detoxify and variations in how much waste your thyroid concentrates, determines how selective its concentrating pump is. This differs from person to person within a family but the traits remain common among family members. Then the next step after the susceptibility is the exposure and merely being around some waste can build this up. In addition, many wastes are beginning to appear on this list. I see papers weekly and usually they have found something new that can also be associated with triggering thyroid disease. If you can name it – it probably can do it.

The first and best documented is perchlorate that forms in the soils, and is a rather common trigger of thyroid disease as we actually have plenty of that in our soils in the Southwest. Fluoride is another common trigger for thyroid disease, as it is added to the municipal waters in many areas. Although some cities are reconsidering and may possibly be decreasing its usage, it is still in the water supply in most metropolitan areas. Therefore, the exposure means that these wastes build up inside the thyroid when someone is genetically susceptible, these wastes create a low amount of inflammation, almost like a scratchy irritation going on at a molecular level inside the gland, and it is creating free radical damage.

Then usually there is some triggering event and is most commonly an infection. It can also be a big shift in hormone levels. Therefore, infections or hormonal shifts are often the triggers and that could be a respiratory infection, a bladder infection, a sinus infection. The hormonal swings – the most common one is pregnancy but also any big change such as when menstrual cycles start or when they stop – so we call that menarche or menopause – the first or the last menstrual cycles can also be common triggering mechanisms that make the complete autoimmune process start. Now, you have the three events that go together are the susceptibility, the toxins, and then the final instigating trigger.

So how do we prevent this and can we prevent this? Well, we cannot 100% prevent it but some steps can certainly lower your odds of getting it and one of the biggest ones comes back to iodine again. You want adequate but not excessive iodine. They call iodine the "Goldilocks mineral" – not too hot and not too cold but you need to get it just right – especially true for your thyroid function.

Moreover, how do you do that? Well, it is not too difficult. You want to use iodized salt for your home cooking, and then primarily eat home cooking. The salt conundrum is that we are consuming much too much salt and it is having a big effect on our health. The Center for Disease Control, a few years ago, estimated that if they could only reduce the American salt intake by one teaspoon per person per day over a year that would translate to 90,000 lives saved annually – so 90,000 fewer people would die per year if we could all go down by one teaspoon of salt per day. Powerful stuff – amazing stuff. In addition, we often focus on the wrong things as dangers. That is one of our biggest dangers and we do not think about it as so deadly.

However, the paradox here is that with getting too much salt we are generally not getting iodized salt. Whenever we have salt in a ready-made food, packaged at a supermarket, or served at a restaurant, that salt does not contain iodine. The expectation when iodine fortification policies were put in place was that people would be consuming the bulk of their salt from foods made at home and that it was not necessary to be included in processed foods and that it could result as the wrong amount. So it is been left out of processed foods. Now we do not eat much homemade food anymore, generally. We eat a lot more of our food from pre-made foods or from restaurant foods. Therefore, we are inching towards being iodine deficient and so far, it is not enough of a problem to where policies have been changed. It does affect about 16-20% of pregnant women. They can get too little. They do have greater needs because they have a separate life growing inside them. Therefore, for your overall health and for the health of your thyroid, do not eat too many processed foods. Mostly have homemade foods and with the food that you eat at home, use iodized salt.

Now the question always comes up among health conscious people – an excellent question – "Well, what about sea salt?" I personally do like sea salt better because primarily it is has about 3% magnesium. It does have other minerals too but the amounts that it has are small enough to be trivial and not useful or effective. However, there is that 3% magnesium – if you are getting most of your salt from sea salt and you are getting a typical (and substantial) amount. That can be as much as a few hundred milligrams of magnesium per day and we can get low in magnesium so it is helpful to have extra amounts of it. I do like sea salt better. Sea salt is often not iodized but you can find iodized versions readily. They are not hard to come across, and are an easy way to help make up for it and keep your thyroid healthy.

Other ways to get adequate iodine are to eat at home and use iodized salt. The better multivitamins contain between fifty and one-hundred micrograms of iodine. If you do not have thyroid disease and you are not on thyroid replacement, it is a good idea to take a multi that has a small amount of iodine as well. If you have thyroid disease, you are better off taking an iodine-free multi. Moreover, with those steps you are healthy. You are going to have adequate amounts and that will lower your rate of getting the disease.

Now other steps are avoiding your exposure to some big thyroid toxins. A common controllable one is mercury, where we are exposed in two primary areas – dental amalgams and seafood. Dental amalgams – you know whether you have them and they are at all due for replacing, by all means replace them with non-metal materials. Moreover, they have become much better nowadays. They have good porcelains and ceramics that are quite durable and stable and are much, much less toxic. If you have a mouthful of metals, taking it out just because – well, that actually releases mercury in your system. So if you are doing that and you need to, it is intelligent to work with a doctor that can also help you with mercury detox so all those things being drilled out will not find their way into your thyroid and your brain, which is where the mercury would go otherwise.

Now with seafood – a difficult question because seafood is extremely healthy. Reams of data state that we are healthier if we have fish regularly. Therefore, it is good for us to have. However, it is intelligent to be conscious of which types of fish have the most mercury. In addition, you can see some good sources such as the FDA or one that I like a lot – the Environmental Working Group, EWG.org. They issue lists of mercury content in fish – high, medium, low. Most high-mercury fish are those you would not be eating daily anyway, such as swordfish, thresher shark, tile fish, or things a little more exotic, so you want to avoid them as a rule.

Now the biggest problem with mercury in seafood is tuna. Tuna is not a high mercury fish. Usually, it is going to be a moderate type level. However, the problem with tuna is that many of us can just eat it every day. During college I probably averaged at least one can of tuna a day for a few years – no kidding. Talking to people over time, I have learned I am not the only one who has done that. Tuna is cheap. It is relatively tasty. It is quite nutritious. It is portable enough. Therefore, it is a handy protein source of many people. However, if you have too much of it the mercury from it does build up. Mercury from seafood is even more toxic than mercury from things like batteries or thermometers or from dental amalgams because it is bound with proteins and it stores in your body more readily. Therefore, it is stuck deep in your tissues, especially your thyroid gland. Therefore, do not have that frequently. Most consider a few servings a month to be safe but you would not want to go above that.

Now another big controllable toxin is fluoride and one more reason not to drink unprocessed tap water. I am not a fan of bottled water but the best thing to do is just have a home filtration unit. Have a reverse osmosis system at home and use purified water that comes from the tap first but has some way to process it to take out the things like the fluoride. Bottled water is quite unregulated, as there are no real governing bodies to say what it can and cannot have and how it is tested. Usually, it is just municipal water put into plastic. So it is often more toxic than you get out of the tap.

So use tap water but have some purification mechanism – at the least, a good filter. Some of the better filters you can read about, they will remove the fluoride and many other compounds. The better way to go is to have a home reverse osmosis system, and these work well. Many bigger cities have companies that rent these to you and the handy thing is that they will do all the care and upkeep and this is often cheaper than it is to just... even for the annual cost of the care alone because you have to replace the filters at least twice a year so consider home reverse osmosis and look at some rental programs as cost-effective, easy ways to do that – a good way to keep fluoride and many other wastes out of your body.

With that, general green living is helpful. Do avoid pesticide sprays inside your house. Outside may not be a big factor but definitely avoid inside the house. An intelligent thing to do too is take your shoes off before you get in the house. Many cultures would be just freaked out if you walked into their home wearing your shoes and it is general cultural stigma not to do that. When we look at toxicology, it becomes an intelligent idea. Most of the waste we are exposed to are from things we track into our house – things like lead or contaminants – they come onto our shoes from the environment and we walk on streets and sidewalks and on ground. We walk that into the house and from there it off-gases and we breathe it in and it enters our bodies. So taking your shoes off before you come into the house makes a considerable difference.

Another big thing about this is minimizing current exposure. Your body has wastes that it is always trying to get rid of. Unfortunately, the bulk of those wastes, they get right back in your bloodstream before they leave in your intestinal tract. The easy way around that is to make your poop as green as you can – and I do not mean food coloring after it is already out. What you want to do is have a high intake of chlorophyll rich green foods. My personal favorite is spinach, and there is much data on that as an excellent thing to help detoxification. The more you can have green foods throughout the day, the better you are going to detox. As I am making this book, I am sipping on some water and I have liquid chlorophyll added to it. It is a good drink with a subtle, gentle taste to it and the chlorophyll itself – good stuff – is the green pigment that helps trap more wastes in our stool and not reabsorb back into our bloodstream.

The other powerful thing to have in a diet is fiber. Any kind of fiber can help but a considerable body of data has shown that the fiber from rice is probably one of the most powerful things for detoxing. Therefore, rice bran is a useful thing to add to the diet. It is tasty. It has a pleasant, nutty flavor and you can add a tablespoon or so to your hot cereal. It is pleasant and it does a good job at helping your body detoxify.

Now if someone has thyroid disease or they have symptoms of early loss of memory, odd movements or tics or changes in personality it is not a bad thing to think about screening for environmental toxins. You want to keep things out and you want to lower your burden but some may actually have enough to where they need some detailed screening done. The screening can be done in several ways. You can test toxins in the blood. You can test toxins in the hair and you can test them in the urine and in the fat tissue. Well the fat tissue is probably the most accurate but it is not practical. I have a scar from when I have done that test before. It takes a rather large volume of tissue for correct reading. However, much of our waste does finish in the fat or the brain.

If we test the urine randomly, it is not super accurate for long-term exposure because the wastes we are most worried about – they do not spontaneously leave your body. They are stuck deeper in your stores. Therefore, we often do a urine test in which we give a provocation and that means we give a dose of medicine that pulls wastes out of your body, then we do a measurement of the urine and we figure out how much came out. We compare that with how much provocation was given, we also factor in the person's size, age, gender, and how active their kidneys were then. All that data together lets us know what is in the body's deeper stores, and you can get a good sense of what toxins could be inside the thyroid, inside the brain or elsewhere.

Now blood tests are also available. The most common ones, such as a serum lead or serum mercury tests, are useful to gauge your short-term exposure. They are handy if you want to know whether you are being exposed on the job. You can do a serum test on a Friday. Compare that with a serum test done first thing on a Monday and you can see the difference and the difference would be your week's long accumulation. I do not use those too much for these purposes because they do not show your lifelong burden and often the biggest question we ask is, "Over the span of your life up to this point, how much waste has built up inside your body?" as it is the principal concern we have.

Hair tests are also available. Hair tests – the good thing is that they are non-invasive. You can do these on yourself at home. Depending on your cutting skills, you may want someone to help you. However, it takes a small amount of hair – so no real trauma – and they can accurately measure many toxins. The problem is that the number of toxins in the hair may not reflect what is in your body. Generally, a correlation is there, but not a tight correlation.

I almost think about the hair test not so much to quantify or count what you have but if someone does it, it is kind of useful to say whether you have toxins in general. If no significant numbers of toxins occur in the hair, there is probably not much in your body. If some toxins show up in your hair, there are probably some in your body but it is difficult to say exactly which and how much. You might have a high level of mercury in your hair but only a small amount in your body or you may have a low amount of aluminum in your hair but actually a high amount in your body. So the hair tests – I do not use them much but if someone has done them I will look at them and if I find nothing there I would not suspect them of carrying toxins in their body. However, if there were findings on the hair test then I would do a detailed test to see if they do have toxins and if so, how much and what type.

Chapter Summary

Hashimoto's Thyroiditis is a disease of the immune system. It comes about in response to chronic thyroid inflammation and eventually breaks down the thyroid gland. Some genetic strains of people are more susceptible to thyroid inflammation than others. This is why thyroid disease clusters in families. Thyroid disease can be prevented to some degree by avoiding toxins and getting adequate but not excessive iodine.

Action Steps

1. Learn to reduce your daily exposure to environmental toxins.

2. Use iodized salt and avoid salt from processed foods such as restaurant food and prepackaged foods.

3. Encourage early screening for thyroid function for family members who are at risk for thyroid disease.

Chapter 2

Ins and Outs of Hashimotos'

Chapter at a Glance

- Differentiating Hypothyroidism from Hashimoto's

- Conventional Diagnostic Process

- Ideal Diagnostic Process

- Normal vs Optimal Labs, Overview

- Conventional Treatment Process

- Ideal Treatment Process

Patients often know that they have hypothyroidism but might not know whether they have Hashimoto's. Others may suspect a form of thyroid disease but have not been diagnosed with it. The question that comes up often is "How is Hashimoto's Disease diagnosed?"

In response, there are two answers – one is the way done today in conventional medicine, and the other is the way it should be done.

The way it is commonly done is for first, someone develops symptoms. These can go on for many, many years. Between ten and twenty years is common. These symptoms are reported to doctors and ideally, they would then be screened for thyroid function. Sometimes they are not even screened but told they have depression or are merely overeating. Other times they are screened but they only have a TSH level drawn. Thyroid disease can go on for some time before the TSH finally moves outside range and reaches the attention of conventional doctors. Many doctors will not treat until the TSH moves well above range or until the T4 levels start to drop. In common practice, when the TSH does elevate above range, most doctors do at least initiate treatment or refer for further evaluation. So that is the point at which treatment is started. Again, if the thyroid function is even checked, it is still common for these symptoms to show up as weight gain, mood changes, or fatigue, and unfortunately, it is all too common that doctors might not even check for thyroid function. An ideal scenario would be that all people would be screened regularly for thyroid function. This could be done more frequently for those with a suspicious family history or pertinent symptoms. By screening, that would be evaluation of their thyroid structure, function, and immunity. Structure here means examination of the gland and ultrasound if the examination was suspicious. Function meaning the actual thyroid output – the TSH, then free levels of T3 and free levels of T4. Immunity meaning evaluation of their body's immunity against the thyroid.

For function, T3 and T4 are checked in two ways. They can be checked either by the total when you are checking if the test only says T4 or T3, or they can also have the free number of the hormones measured. The hormones T3 and T4 are proteins. They are transported throughout your blood by carrier proteins. The amount permanently bound to proteins is inactivated. However, some hormone is not bound and it is free and able to do work. Therefore, when total T4 or T3 are measured, what that means is the total amount of the hormone. That is the combination of the free, the active fraction, plus the bound, inactive fraction.

For most people the amount of active hormone will be an expected percentage of the total hormone. However, often the amount of active hormone is greater or lower than is typical, therefore the total amount of hormone read alone can be misleading. So it is preferred to measure the free amount of the T3 and the T4 as it is the active amount of the hormone – the amount actually doing the work.

Therefore, the ideal workup would start even before symptoms. It would start when there is a strong family history. Now commonly this ideal workup would be started at the point of symptoms and any unusual changed symptoms, it should be worth a screening. That is not to say that the thyroid is the cause of all medical issues. One should also evaluate many other possible causes of symptoms. However, thyroid disease should be on the radar. Because this does affect every cell in the body, no real symptom can be tied to thyroid. Even so, some symptoms are much more probable than others, much more commonly found with thyroid disease than others are.

With symptoms, here is something that is somewhat counterintuitive. You may have seen the long lists of commonly reported thyroid symptoms. These can include symptoms such as the hoarseness of voice, difficulty swallowing, unexplained weight gain, fatigue, dry skin, dry hair, dry nails, muscle pain, depression, anxiety, constipation, cold intolerance.

People rarely have many of those symptoms at once. Although they can be severe, it is not common to have many of them. The most common number statistically, is between two and four.

I will be talking to someone about the symptoms and say, "With the weight gain – have you had the dry skin? Have you had the hair loss? Have you had the constipation?" and people often will say, "Well no, I don't have those symptoms" and they often believe that if they do not have all those other symptoms, and then they do not have thyroid disease. However, it does not work that way. It is much more typical that people have a distinct set of a few symptoms, but they do not have the others. I almost think of it like a deck of cards, and you have about a dozen cards with big symptoms and everybody receives a few cards differing from one another. Not everyone therefore has the same symptom profile with thyroid disease.

In the ideal workup, other causes should also be considered. These can include blood sugar disturbances, adrenal disease, anemia, and kidney problems. A thorough laboratory workup, a good physical examination can show if any of these other factors are present.

Hashimoto's Disease is a different condition from many other diseases in that it is not something you can readily diagnose without actually taking someone's thyroid out and completely mincing it. Doctor Hashimoto – he defined it as a set of changes that occur, which you can evaluate under a microscope. So when you have all or part of someone's gland under a microscope you can see the changes occurring and there are many markers we use that help us assume that it is occurring less invasively. It is not convenient to remove everyone's thyroid when you are suspicious of it so we do things such as blood tests and examinations. Therefore, because of that, there is no one thing that says you do not have it. It is a matter of receiving enough data to see whether that is so. In addition, that should include examinations of the gland's structure. That is important both to confirm why the symptoms are occurring but also because if it is the cause then there is a greater risk for structural problems and the primary things there are nodules and the risk towards cancer.

Therefore, if someone does have an inflammatory disease against their thyroid, they do have a higher risk for developing thyroid cancer and because of that, it is important to be regular with evaluation of the gland. Moreover, two ways are used, by either physical examination or ultrasound. Both are actually helpful. The good thing about physical examination is you can have a quick once-over of the size, structure, and the quality of the gland. Often, that alone is helpful to gauge how one is responding to treatment, how the gland is coming down in size as it should. The ultrasound is the most critical for identifying any abnormalities because you can obtain an accurate size on them, down to the millimeter. That is excellent for tracking abnormalities such as nodules or calcifications. If these things remain in the same location and at the same size from one ultrasound to the next, we feel more confident that they are not cancerous.

It is common to have nodules, for those who have thyroid disease. In addition, with the nodules, it is important to track them repeatedly to know whether they are changing. Generally, if they are within specific size parameters or a specific location, and their size is not shifting, they are benign. They are rather harmless. However, it is important to obtain a good evaluation of those. The other good thing about an ultrasound is that you cannot always identify nodules from physical examination. They have shown that the best doctors, who do physical examinations, will pick up nodules on about 5% of the population but if you take the same population and do ultrasounds on everyone, you are going to discover that 20% might have nodules. Therefore, ultrasounds are more sensitive and they are more accurate. The examinations are a convenient tool that the doctor can do easily without time or expense, but regular ultrasounds are important.

Therefore, an ideal workup would involve physical examination, ultrasound, detailed blood tests, and that is how the disease can be caught at its earliest stages when the symptoms are first showing. Unfortunately, it is common that those steps are not taken. Often even those who have been identified as having the disease are not given proper evaluation of the structure of the gland. They are not being monitored to see if they have nodules, if the nodules are growing at all.

Then the question arises – "Well, why is there this big gap? Why is it that so many people have this condition but it's not checked thoroughly and not addressed at early stages?" and there is probably not one simple answer but what tends to shift and shape medical practice is procedures and new medications. You can show that in one county, if the reimbursement rate for a C-section is $3,000 and in the next county the rate for the C-section is $2,000, one county will do more C-sections. This has been shown repeatedly. Even further, if the counties reverse their reimbursement schedule to where the first county pays less and the second county pays more, the rate of C-sections flips. So it is probably not a conscious change but medical practices are changed by procedures. Therefore, if there are doctors of high-end procedures gravitating towards them, and because not many high-end procedures are involved with thyroid disease, there is not much doctors can do repeatedly to be paid a fair amount. So they do not have much investment in spending time with people and working out their symptoms and helping them recover when there is not going to be procedures involved with it.

Now the other thing that does drive medicine is newer medications. Doctors' habits are strongly driven by marketing. It is no mystery that pharmaceutical companies do this often. Almost any new medication that comes out is not a new treatment. It is rather just a slight modification on an old treatment and it is usually no better. Now there may be subtle differences but usually there is not a significant change between the new medicine and the old medicine that it is replacing.

However, because the new medicines are outside the reach of patents, they have typically anywhere from five to twenty times the cost factor associated with them so they are much more expensive. In addition, because of this price burden the companies have to market the new medications aggressively to doctors to encourage them to use them. Moreover, this works. This does have a clear influence on prescribing practices. Even little things as seemingly innocuous as carrying a pen with a drug name will cause you to write more scripts for that drug, and there is just no way around that. Something being in your present consciousness has a big effect on your practices and what you are going to do. Therefore, these things make a difference.

With thyroid disease there are no fancy, new medications. The medicines we are using now have been around for literally one hundred years. In addition, honestly, we do not need radical advances. We could improve somewhat in our medications but basically, with replacement medicines, we need things that will approximate what your body would make anyway and we do have good versions of that, especially with a desiccated thyroid. We will talk more in detail about medications and what might be an ideal medicine, but overall there has been nothing new for some time and because of that there is no big excitement and no big push for doctors to be involved. That is the biggest reason why there is a big gap. The sad fact is that in the institutions that focus on thyroid disease such as The American Thyroid Association, all these things I am saying about early diagnosis and treatment and the effects of it are all well-known but these things have not affected day-to-day medical practice.

A big gap remains between those data points and what doctors do regularly in general practice or even often in endocrinology.

Then the next step would be treatment – how is this condition treated? Just as I described for diagnosis, I will talk about the typical treatment scenario and the ideal treatment scenario as well.

The typical scenario is that treatment is started after someone has been diagnosed and that diagnosis often does come late. For many it does not come at all because doctors are only looking at a late stage of the illness. So treatment is also based – in the conventional guidelines – on a few variables.

They look at the normal range of the TSH and the T4 levels and that is it. Moreover, the treatment is T4 replacement, that means levothyroxine – generic name for Synthroid – and that is the most common thyroid treatment given. Now policy guidelines by The American Academy of Clinical Endocrinology and The American Academy of Family Practitioners is that this is all that you need to give T4-only medications. If you dig deep into policies they will say whether patients are intensely symptomatic still and you test them more thoroughly and find they are low in T3 you could include a T3-based medicine such as Cytomel, allowed in rare cases but is not commonly used and then only for a big suppression in T3.

Therefore, the goal of treatment is the normalization of the TSH, and the TSH – that is our pituitary asking the thyroid to work – becomes a backward indicator. When the thyroid is pushing out too little hormones, the TSH elevates. If there are too many hormones the TSH goes down. So by giving T4 replacement the TSH does tend to decrease. In addition, in the body, the TSH is strongly regulated by the T4 and that is because in your system, you do make primarily T4. However, you also do make T3, and when you are healthy, you are going to have T3 and T2 made by the rest of your body out of the T4. Therefore, in your system, if you have enough T4 and things are working right, you are generally okay on the other hormones. Yet when you have thyroid disease, this conversion does not always work right. That is because there is some problem with the thyroid function, and then there is a much higher rate of poor utilization of T4. Although T4 may push down the TSH and may normalize it, people still can be lacking the T3 or the T2 levels.

In addition, the other big issue is that the goal of replacement therapy to push down TSH is to push TSH back into the normal range. We will talk more about this but the difficulty with the normal range is it is normal for the range of people who have been tested with it and that is mostly people that have thyroid disease. People that have no thyroid symptoms, no known disease, and no family history – they are not going to be having thyroid tests done often – not often at all. However, those who do have thyroid disease, especially those who have the most difficulty and the most symptoms – they are going to be tested the most often and they have a big impact on where that normal range plays out.

Because of that, the normal range we go by now is 0.4-4.5, if we did look at the healthiest population that did not have any continuing thyroid issues, that range would come way down to 0.3-1.5 and because of that many people are on the upper end of that normal range – between the 1.5 and the 4.5 – they might still be symptomatic. Moreover, by current guidelines they are in the normal range. They are at the endpoint of treatment, and there is no real discussion or standards for what to do with them after that point and if they are symptomatic. The guidelines do not call for looking more deeply or changing their medication. Though many people are on T4-only medications, they may not be receiving good amounts of T3 or T2 out of the deal, and they may have their TSH in that upper end of the normal range, between 1.5 and 4.5, and in those categories, they can be symptomatic. They can still be suffering significantly. Sometimes, they can have the identical symptoms to the same degree they had when they were first diagnosed. So a quick summary – the treatment, by the current conventional model, is only for a T4 replacement and only to move the TSH back into the normal range. Often, the other hormones are not looked at or not evaluated.

In contrast, what would the ideal treatment strategy look like? Well, the treatment should have several goals, the most important of which would be restoring ideal levels of the hormones. Another critical goal would be establishing a healthy structure of the thyroid and evaluating that. Again, people who have thyroid disease stand the greatest risk for thyroid cancer. Thyroid cancer is the fastest increasing type of cancer in America today so it needs to be taken much, much more seriously.

The other goal of treatment is to assure that people have healthy immune systems, meaning that they do not have a real active, continuing attack against their thyroid or against other portions of their body. Autoimmune diseases tend to congregate. If you have one, you have a greater chance of having others and the more poorly controlled the autoimmune disease, the more likely you are to have poor control or new onset of other autoimmune disease. The more likely others are to pop up when one is poorly controlled. Immune regulation is one of those too.

In addition, probably the most important goal would just be the health and the well-being of the patient. The sad fact is that in the conventional guidelines that is irrelevant. Clearly, the treatment goals state that the one outcome of treatment is normalization of the TSH.

I saw a cartoon a while ago. It showed a stereotypical older, pudgy, bald doctor in a white lab coat behind a desk and he was reviewing an obvious x-ray. In the x-ray, you could see the skull and the ribs and whatever. In addition, sitting across the desk from him apparently was the patient and the doctor was looking at this x-ray saying, "Well I can't figure out what's wrong with you. Your x-ray looks perfectly fine."" The doctor was looking at the x-ray but not looking at the patient. Had he done so he would have seen that the patient was actually a skeleton, just as the skeleton on the x-ray. So obviously, this person was not well. They were nothing but bones. However, according to what the doctor saw on his test there were no problems. Moreover, that was an extreme example of what happens in medicine.

When you become so fixated on our data points, our tests, and our technology we often forget that the point is to alleviate suffering and improve health, which should be the highest goal for thyroid treatment but unfortunately by policy, the sole goal is normalization of the TSH. In addition, if you are gaining weight and you are depressed and miserable who cares what the piece of paper says? That is of no consolation at all. Therefore, the real goal is restoration of full health. Moreover, as we go about these we will talk about all those steps in detail. I will give a quick summary of each.

The first, as far as the establishment of normal hormone levels – now that should consider the TSH, the Free T3, the Free T4 – and that also should consider other relevant nutrients involved with these hormones being formed and converted. This includes many key minerals and a few relevant vitamins and these levels should be brought back to ideal ranges – not just broad population average ranges.

With thyroid disease, it is also intelligent to consider the other portions of the endocrine system. The complete endocrine glandular network is connected. The old song – "the leg bone's connected to the knee bone" – well that is true here too. The thyroid is connected to the adrenals and the adrenals are connected to the ovaries and they are all connected to the pituitary and the hypothalamus, and if you have testicles, they are connected. So all these things do tie in and do relate.

When one gland has been shown to have a disease it is common that the other glands have had to alter their function because of this and they have had to work harder, work differently and sometimes they can start to decompensate and not work as well just because of the strain they had by taking on changes from the thyroid. Therefore, this should evaluate all the body's glands and all their outputs, and they should be brought back to ideal ranges.

The next step, as far as concerns the structure of the gland, is regular examinations and ultrasounds. In addition, if there are suspicious, abnormal findings there may be a call for biopsies or further evaluation or treatment. An ultrasound should be done at least annually and if they are abnormal or changing, more often can be appropriate. Therefore, that is the other stage of this.

Now the immune portion – there should be initial screening for a big variety of autoimmune diseases. This would include celiac, lupus, rheumatoid arthritis, scleroderma, Sjogren's Disease. Some simple blood markers can do these. Therefore, when the patient is first diagnosed as having Autoimmune Hashimoto's Thyroiditis they should also be evaluated for having related autoimmune diseases and if there are abnormalities showing up there, these things should also be given due, appropriate, specific treatment, then also reassessed and tracked.

If the patient is stable and you are feeling well, healthy, and you are meeting your goals, it would not require as detailed, continuing screening for other autoimmune issues, but if your health is not where you want it to be or if it is shifting – if it was stable, then shifts to a poor condition – then it would be intelligent to go back and refresh to see whether there has been any shift, and see if there has been any new onset autoimmune reactions because that can happen.

In addition, with the immune component, it is also beneficial to see early whether there are stressors on the immune system. Moreover, the two largest categories of immune stressors would be allergies and infections.

Allergies come in several types such as airborne, dietary, acute, and chronic. In addition, acute allergies are just that – they hit you quickly and cause immediate symptoms. The chronic ones might not act as quickly but tend to cause more continuing, persistent, problematic symptoms that may not always be obviously paired with exposure. This means that you can breathe something or eat something and because the onset of symptoms is gradual continuing for a while, it may not be apparent that the thing you were just exposed to was the trigger.

So the chronic allergies – they can be less obvious and it is common that we will see someone with thyroid disease and screen them for allergies and they may say, "Well, but I don't have allergies." Most people think about receiving a bad rash from eating peanuts or having sniffles every spring when the hay fever comes around but it is more than that. People can have just continuing, chronic, low-grade symptoms like fatigue or muscle pains or aches or digestive issues and they may not be different from one day to the next and this can be related to allergies, especially from the chronic, hidden food allergies. Therefore, that is an intelligent part of the initial screening as well.

The chronic infections – this is relevant to some more than others, but there are those who carry low-grade, continuing infections in their body that are not completely resolved. In addition, the more things your immune system is attacking, the more aggressive your immune system becomes. If it is also prone to attack your thyroid, the level of attack will be worsened based on the amount and the severity of other infections you are carrying at a given time. Now certainly some infections are obvious, like having a cold or flu. Others such as the chronic allergies can also be less apparent. Some big ones that fall in this category would be chronic, low-grade fungal sinusitis. Usually, someone will have some degree of continuing sinus symptoms.

Another common thing we will see is chronic Epstein Barr virus infection. This is a virus to which the majority of us have been exposed, and like most people, we have it, then we suppress it, keep it turned off, and it does not affect us. Some suffered with it badly enough to where they were diagnosed as having mononucleosis, most commonly earlier in life, but most people never have it severe enough so it becomes diagnosed as being nothing different from just a cold or flu. So most people have had it but a subset of people do not completely shut it off and they have like a mild, continuing flu persistently. We suspect this more, especially if someone has low-grade, intermittent fevers, unexplained, recurrent sore throat, swollen lymph nodes or if they are just prone to become sick easily.

The other big category of chronic infections would be intestinal. A common one people know about with this would be candidiasis. This is a real thing. A big variety of organisms live in the intestinal tract and most of them are just along for the ride. They are harmless. A few of them are actually helpful to our immune systems and our nutrient formation and they are important to us, then a few are harmful if they can be so. That is what yeast is. Various strains of yeast occur in the intestinal tract but candida receives the most attention. If we have situations that weaken our good, protective bacteria then the yeast – the candida – can merely overgrow and become more aggressive and harmful.

A common condition that causes this would be the continual use of antibiotics – taking antibiotics several times per year or for longer periods such as for acne for children or even as adults. However, longer or recurrent courses of antibiotics are common triggers for that. Now another thing that can do this is the continual use of oral contraceptives – birth control pills. They do act similarly to weak antibiotics and they do slow the growth of your healthful bacteria so they can also make you more likely to develop yeast overgrowth over time.

Aside from that, another trigger for yeast can be a high intake of processed grains, white flour products, or sugar in the diet. Nowadays you do not need to look too hard to find cases of this. Many people do intake too much of those foods, and the organisms that grow in your intestinal tract depend on the kind of food put into your intestinal tract. It is like a big compost pile. If you have ever had a compost pile you have learned that some things just cannot go in it or it will ruin the organisms in there and that is what sugar does to our gut flora. It hurts the good bacteria but stimulates the yeast excessively. Over time, the yeast gains such a foothold and becomes so pervasive that it shifts the chemistry to make the complete intestinal tract a better place for it but a worse place for your good bacteria, and that becomes a vicious circle. The yeast can create some localized symptoms of discomfort – gas, bloating, and irregularity – but it can also weaken your immune system and becoming a chronic, low-grade, infectious stressor.

Therefore, a good workup would look at these other stressors on the immune system as well.

Moreover, with well-being and symptoms, the best workups and treatments would closely evaluate that person's health and involve where it was before it started, where it could be ideally and map out "What are the key symptoms? What are the key barriers?" then be sure to take all the steps to restore things to their ideal levels.

Chapter Summary

The Majority of people with hypothyroidism in the modern world have Hashimoto's Thyroiditis. This can be the case even if your tests for thyroid antibodies are negative.

Most conventional doctors diagnose hypothyroidism solely on a TSH elevated above range and a T4 or free T4 below range.

Hashimoto's Thyroiditis can be present and causing negative effects long before the TSH elevates above range and the T4 or free T4 goes below range. The disease can be detected at earlier stages by measuring antibodies, performing thyroid ultrasounds, comparing lab values against optimal ranges and by considering pertinent symptoms.

Most conventional doctors treat hypothyroidism with T4 (levothyroxine, common brand: Synthroid) therapy only with the goal of reducing the TSH to the normal range. Many who have completed this still have hypothyroid symptoms.

People with Hashimoto's Thyroiditis get the most benefit when the triggers of their disease are identified and corrected and their blood levels reflect those of the disease-free populations.

Action Steps

4. If you suspect thyroid disease but have not been diagnosed, have a thyroid ultrasound done and comprehensive thyroid labs including TSH, free T4, free T3, antithyroperoxidase antibodies, antithyroglobulin antibodies, thyroglobulin and reverse T3.

5. Work with a doctor or educate your doctor about optimal vs normal values for thyroid lab values.

Chapter 3

Optimize Your Dose

Chapter At a Glance

- Getting your dose right is one of the most important steps you can take to feel better and to lower long term health risks.

- Optimal TSH

- Types of Thyroid Medicine

- Role of T2

- Natural Desiccated Thyroid for Hashimoto's?

- Too much can feel like too little

- Understanding free T4 and free T3 - peripheral control

- Reverse T3

Getting your thyroid dosing right. This is an important topic for feeling your best. So often, you do hear that thyroid replacement does not take care of all the symptoms. Yet it is a big factor. So often people who feel that replacement has not worked for them have not been on the right types or the right amounts. Commonly the dosing used is based only on either reference ranges – as in the conventional model – or it is based only on symptoms – as in the alternative model. Moreover, both have their shortcomings.

Briefly, the reference ranges we talked about in more detail are established from averages for the population being tested and the population being tested for thyroid disease mostly is the population that has thyroid disease. Roughly, 85% of those who have thyroid blood tests already have a diagnosis of having hypothyroidism and they are being monitored for dose adjustment purposes. Roughly, another 10% have suspicious symptoms they are being evaluated for and perhaps 5% are people that have good thyroid function, that are just having random screening tests done. So the ranges are biased toward the diseased population. Therefore, with the conventional model, dosing is stopped once TSH scores are back inside the normal range and for that reason, many people have a thyroid function unlike healthy people's thyroid function.

The TSH represents how much your body is asking for from your thyroid. So the more hormone that your gland is making, the lower the TSH will become. This holds true for the hormone your gland would make but it is equally true for hormones that you would be taking if you were being given replacement therapy. So TSH – it is a good indicator but it is a backward indicator. With what you make or what you are taking, the higher numbers represent less thyroid activity and the lower numbers represent more thyroid activity.

So commonly, the alternative medicine world will discredit the TSH. This is throwing the baby out with the bathwater. The TSH is an accurate test. It does represent your body's overall thyroid hormone balance. However, the shortcoming as it has been used is that it is attached to ranges that do not reflect ideal thyroid function.

One of the bigger studies on this was done in Turkey. They started with hundreds of people. Then they took out everyone that had known thyroid disease, possible thyroid disease based upon symptoms, strong family histories of thyroid disease, medications that could skew thyroid function or pregnancy.

The remaining people had no variables that should have skewed their thyroid function. They had no factors that should have affected that. Therefore, the remaining people were then tested several times over several months to check how their thyroid function scores were and it was fascinating. The variation in that population was extremely small. What also showed up was that the variation from person to person – meaning how different Joe's scores were from Sue's scores – were no greater than the variation from one person to themselves – meaning how much variation there was between Susie's scores on Day 1, Day 10 and Day 30 of the test.

So the variation from one person to the next with the variation from one person to themselves were about the same and the TSH showed the biggest difference in this study from the ranges that we consider normal for it. In this study, no one had TSH scores greater than 1.5, which was shocking. In addition, there was a strong median score – strong average score – at roughly 0.99. Therefore, 1 – or just a tad below 1 – is about where the TSH levels are in the healthiest population, with a small amount of expected and acceptable variation.

In the conventional thyroid tests, they still call normal up to 4.5 because the score is an average of those who have had mostly thyroid disease. One of the biggest first steps is to bring your TSH back down to a healthy range. So many people that have been diagnosed as hypothyroid and are on treatment are not feeling well and their TSH might be 2.5 or 3.5 or 4.2 and by many conventional guidelines they are said to be fine yet it is easy understanding why they would be symptomatic with levels like that. They are much more hypothyroid than someone in the healthiest of the populations would be and that alone is a big source of symptoms. One of the first steps to making yourself feel better is bringing your TSH back down to a healthy range and I will talk a little about various medications here.

Now we can loosely categorize those into synthetic and natural forms of thyroid. By synthetic, we mean things that have been synthesized – made in a factory. The synthetic versions of thyroid hormones are actually chemically identical to the hormones the body makes. The variation is not significant. Something that I have found rather ironic is that in natural medicine we pride ourselves in the use of natural hormones when doing hormone replacement therapy. Yet with thyroid treatment, what we would call a natural hormone by the same definition is now called a synthetic. Therefore, if Synthroid were a chemical used for hormone replacement therapy for estrogen, for example, the same logic would call it a natural hormone. Even though it is synthesized, it is synthesized in a chemically identical form.

Therefore, Synthroid and the other synthetics – including levoxyl, levothyroxine, cytomel, and liothyronine – are not bad as such. They are simply partial. They simply lack other hormones. The most active ones are T4, T3, and T2. However, T2 does not receive the attention that it deserves. It is definitely the Rodney Dangerfield in the room. T4 and T3 – those are pre-made medications – Synthroid, brand name, levothyroxine, Levothroid, levoxyl. Those are all different versions of T4-only. For T3 – Cytomel and generic liothyronine, and a combination product called Thyrolar made by Forest Labs, the same people who make Armour thyroid. It is a T4-T3 combination with a 4:1 T4 to T3 ratio. I have used this product occasionally with patients who clearly benefit from T3 but wish to avoid an animal product. However, it is used so seldom that pharmacies often do not stock it or keep adequate supplies to have someone's needs met. Therefore, I do not use it much for that reason especially.

One advantage to having T2 included in your replacement therapy and the only way to consistently receive that in the States is to use desiccated thyroid, which is ground up, freeze-dried pig thyroid. It sounds rather crude – and it is actually been used for thousands of years for these purposes – but it is probably our best approximation of what the human body would make. It does include all the active thyroid proteins – T4, T3, and T2. Some argue that there may be benefit from T1 also. These T numbers mean one molecule of tyrosine (T) plus X-numbers of iodine attached to it. So T4 would be tyrosine, then four iodine atoms, T3 would be tyrosine with three iodine atoms and T2 is tyrosine with two iodine atoms – so a simple process.

However, T2 clearly does have a metabolic benefit. Unfortunately, we have no means of measuring it outside research. No commercial labs do it regularly so we cannot test it. The other problem is that the T2 does not push down the

TSH. The T3 and the T4 – if we give these hormones – they will make the TSH become lower and consequently we have a sense of how much total thyroid hormone that person is taking. T2 does not do that so when it is not there, no alteration in the TSH occurs. The TSH would not be lower because of the person taking a T2 compound but also when T2 is not given and it is lacking, the TSH will not be higher so you will not see that it is missing. Now there were some papers done in the 60s and they showed that if someone did not have a thyroid and they were taking a T4-only medication the amount of T2 that they had would only be about 10% of what it would be for someone making their own thyroid. Moreover, T2 is one of the most important hormones for regulating metabolic rate – the rate at which we burn calories.

When you put all this together and desiccated thyroid looks appealing. You can also take T4 and T3 together and that would be like a Synthroid-Cytomel combo, which is commonly given by conventional doctors trying to go a little outside their box in trying to accommodate their patients, so include some Cytomel. It does still lack the T2. The other advantage desiccated thyroid has over T4 and T3 is because of the proteins, it is metabolized in a slower period. It results as a self-regulating time-release version. The hormones do not enter the bloodstream as quickly whereas T3 medications used in isolation, to make your levels stable you would need more frequent dosing throughout the day. It would not work well to have just once daily dosing. You would have rather substantial variations in your T3 throughout the day. In addition, if you have not realized this already it is difficult to work in a time of day to take something on a completely empty stomach, so imagine trying to take three doses in regularly each day away from food. That would be a difficult battle. So desiccated thyroid looks nice.

Now one thing that comes up a lot is that some people argue those who have Hashimoto's cannot safely take desiccated thyroid. Now whenever I hear that, immediately it tells me that someone has a shallow understanding of hypothyroidism. Hashimoto's causes most of hypothyroidism in America. No perfect numbers are available, but many estimate that it is upward of 95%. So if you are hypothyroid and you have not been told you have Hashimoto's you probably have it anyway. It is much more common than not. I always wonder if someone with Hashimoto's cannot take desiccated thyroid, but who in the world would? Because there are not many others who would need it.

A few papers have looked at this exact topic – how desiccated thyroid affects the immune function. The warning about desiccated thyroid with Hashimoto's goes something like this. People argue that taking thyroid proteins orally somehow will stimulate the antibody production. It will somehow worsen your body's attack on your gland. The little data done on that topic was not recent but there was some good studies done in the 50s and they looked just at that. They looked at how the body's immune function changed for someone with Hashimoto's taking desiccated thyroid compared with someone else taking a synthetic version of thyroid. What happened here was actually a beneficial effect, meaning that taking desiccated thyroid decreased the immune response. It made that person not have as active an immune response against their thyroid. Therefore, if anything, the effect is likely to be positive. It may be one more factor in diminishing antibodies and diminishing the overall immune response – and we will talk about that more too. So desiccated thyroid can safely be taken for those who have Hashimoto's.

I have just scoured medical research databases trying to find the actual origin of the warning saying otherwise. It turns out to be like the telephone game. It has been repeated many times, yet no one seems to know where it started. I can find no basis in fact. The data that I have found has shown the opposite – there can be beneficial effects. Moreover, I certainly see this. I manage thousands of people with Hashimoto's, most of them on desiccated thyroid, and I do not see any consistent problems with it skewing their immune functions. Therefore, if it is something that has concerned you, please do not worry unduly about that.

So back to the overall coarse adjustments – the first step is making the TSH dialed in and by "dialed in" that means for most people lowered to a healthy range if they have been working with a conventional doctor. And the ideal level is going to be right around 0.5 to 1.5 – easy ballpark – somewhere close to 1.0 is ideal. There are concerns raised if someone has had structural thyroid problems and that would be a history of thyroid cancer or a history of nodules or a history of a goiter and those are all cases in which we want the TSH to be as low as reasonably possible – and here is why.

Remember the TSH elevates when the body needs more thyroid hormone. Now what it is actually doing to the gland is stimulating it – thyroid-stimulating hormone. So a little more detail – by "stimulating," that means it causes the thyroid to grow new cells. So if you have got a healthy feedback system and a healthy thyroid, if there were too little hormone coming out your thyroid would be stimulated and it would become bigger and those cells would become a little more active and that growth would then encourage enough extra hormone to compensate for that small lack – and vice versa. If adequate or excessive hormone occurs, the TSH lowers and the normal rate of cell repair would slow, causing a small decrease in the mass of thyroid and a small decrease in the activity of its cells. So that is great.

If there are things you do not want in your thyroid – perhaps a few wayward, leftover cells from thyroid cancer or a nodule or a goiter – you do not want those things growing. You do not want any more of a growth signal on those foreign tissues than you would have to have. The ideal scenario is to keep the TSH well below 1.0 – generally close to 0.5. Now the danger here is that you are going to be up against the edge of there being too much thyroid hormone. Therefore, you are close to a hyperthyroid dose when you are in this range and people strategically kept their TSH on the low end have to be educated about hyperthyroid side effects and complications. They do also have to be monitored rather closely for cardiac issues and bone density changes. Being up against the hyperthyroid side can strain the body in those ways.

The side effects are as if you drank a pot of coffee but you did not drink a pot of coffee. You are wired and over-stimulated and it can last throughout the day. It tends to be not subtle. At first it might be something you may not be clear about but if it is progressed, it is not subtle. You are obviously wired. Your heart rate may be elevated at rest. You may be sweating when everyone else is cold. You could have a tremor and just be anxious and not feeling well. It is generally not subtle when it is happening and it should be addressed. There are some rare cases where people are in that range of 0.5 to 1.0 – they still can have some of those side effects. If they have had complications such as the thyroid cancer or the nodules or the goiters – especially the cancer – there may be a judgment call where the side effects are better to be managed by themselves than the dose reduced. Otherwise it would raise the risk of the cancer recurring or issues worsening. Therefore, that is one situation – if there have been structural problems – then a different, lower TSH is targeted. You want to be on the lowest end of that normal, healthy range. But barring structural issues most do well when it is close to 1.0 – a little above, a little below that – so that becomes the target.

Again, the TSH is backward so if it is above target, the dose should be raised gently and below target, the dose should be lowered. Now dose changes – you do not want them to happen too quickly. Typically, a 10% or so change per two weeks is adequate. The TSH – especially when it is high or low – it is not linear, meaning that above a specific range the numbers could be interchangeable. If your TSH was 7.0 and the next day it was 20.0, after that it was 100, then it was back down to 12 – it does not mean that it changed a lot between those days. It is pegged and your pituitary is yelling, but that yell can be variable. When the scores are jumping around that much, someone would not need a greater dose increase if the TSH was 100 than they would need for a TSH of 20.

Now another factor is that the TSH can take up to three months to level out and reach a steady state. When somebody has been off by a large margin – whether high or low – you promptly want the person back to normal. However, you do have to factor in the period it takes the TSH to level out. So I often will recheck at lower than three-month intervals but I will remember that further drift is possible. So if someone has a high TSH or even say they are 4.0-4.1 and we raised their dosage and a month later they are back down to 1.0, to me that says we have probably overdone it because a further drift is likely in the next couple months and that means they are going to move to the hyperthyroid state. It is okay to check it sooner, your doctor may encourage that, and you may wish that if you are not feeling well but one should remember that short of three months there could be some drift. Therefore, if you hit target fast or you are overshooting it, it is probably going to keep going.

Now here is one area where I have already parted ways with the conventional world by shooting for ideal TSH – not normal TSH – and the funny thing is that is not a parting of the way with the upper echelon of thyroidology by any means. The American Thyroid Association – all statements that I have made are statements that they make regularly. However, it is a parting of the way with conventional practice for general family practitioners, internal medicine doctors and even many endocrinologists. Many still do go by normal ranges or close to it. However, we have hard data saying that ideal ranges are much more meaningful and people do much better at them, and they are safe.

Now the alternative world is the opposite. Their shortcoming is that they tend to over-treat thyroid conditions and they often tend to over-diagnose. Not everyone that has a possible thyroid symptom has thyroid disease. Many do and commonly they are not diagnosed but a shortcoming I see of the alternative world is that people are put on thyroid treatment even if they do not need it. Even if their thyroid was not the actual cause of their symptoms. Then the next issue that I have is people are placed on high doses of thyroid. Many authors have said flat out that even if the TSH is low, it is okay to continue raising doses until symptoms are idealized. Like many of these things, that represents a shallow understanding of how the thyroid works. An additional difficulty is that you can have similar symptoms when your dose is high as you do when your dose is too low. I will go into that in a little more detail here.

All strategies need to consider how much hormone the gland would make if it were working perfectly. This is called physiologic dosing. What I mean is a healthy thyroid is going to make a specific amount of hormone and an adult will only make so much thyroid hormone. Above that, your body will not produce amounts in excess of it. Therefore, when someone is taking doses way above what the body would make – after we factor in any issues of absorption – then you are probably just overdosing. Moreover, what can happen is that a point is reached where thyroid hormones can become a stimulant. They can be no different from cocaine, caffeine, or any other stimulant and there can be a time to where when you take a stimulant, commonly you feel great at first but by definition, the stimulant is not sustainable. That is why we differentiate in herbal medicine, stimulants from tonics. Tonics are things that raise your strength and vitality in a lasting way. Stimulants are things that have a rebound effect, meaning they push you up and you are going to bounce back down. In addition, the thyroid hormone dosages way above what your body would make – they are more stimulants than tonics.

So a common cycle I will see is that someone may be pushed up to say a three grain dose of desiccated thyroid and for a few weeks – boy, the lights just come right back on. They are energized, their weight is coming around, they have cleaned up their garage – they are feeling well and their mood is improved. Then it drops off and it seems so, so intuitive and logical both to the person and to the doctor that "Hey, if we did this before and raised the dose and it worked better why don't we raise the dose again?" I certainly understand that logic. That makes sense. What will happen commonly is that with that next dose increase you are probably going to see the same thing again. You are probably going to see someone doing a little better, and then dropping off again. Now part of the mind process is "Hey, I'm tired and I'm on a high dose and since I'm tired I can't be getting too much and I felt better at first when I raised that dose." Therefore, it seems so obvious that the remedy is to continue raising the dosage. I have had patients that have called me and consulted me from around the country that have been on doses upward of 8 grains or higher.

Now an adult woman's body that does not have a thyroid gland at all is going to require somewhere around 2 grains per day. If that person has a large body mass, they have poor digestive function, and they cannot absorb well, sometimes they will need 2.5 or 3 grains and no more. Managing thousands and thousands of people, I do not think I have anyone who is on greater than a 3-grain dosage and most are on between 1.5 and 2 grains who do not have much of their own internal output. Whenever someone is taking much more than that, they are probably not receiving benefit from it. If we convert that into a dose of Synthroid, that 2-grain dose of desiccated thyroid is roughly 200 micrograms, and similarly, if someone needs more than 200 micrograms they should be switching medicines or seeing what else is wrong.

Now the pitfall involving the fatigue issues is this. Your thyroid is regulated internally and peripherally. By "internally," we mean direct things that act on it such as your pituitary and hypothalamus. Now "peripherally," we mean your liver, your kidneys, your intestinal tract, your detox pathways, your cells – there are many ways your body can control how you use thyroid. It is just so powerful and so important to get it right there is a whole lot of overlap and a whole lot of backup mechanisms. When your dose is a little higher than you need the first thing that happens is of course your body quits asking for as much. The TSH goes lower. Then also the way you eliminate thyroid. The way you break it down into reverse T3, the rate at which you urinate it, the amount of which is bound by sulfation in your intestinal tract. These all start to increase and those are all adaptive mechanisms your body uses to protect itself against poisoning from excessive thyroid. This explains why when you are taking more than you need you are first doing better, then you feel tired again – because your body is dumping it out and is also why someone taking a high dose of thyroid can feel fatigued – because they are eliminating it so quickly. We can see a mix of hyperthyroid complications, and then fatigue symptoms.

Now an important point here too with thyroid dosing is looking at the free hormone and this is something else commonly misunderstood by the alternative medicine world.

The free hormones – they shift after the TSH shifts. Now by "after," I mean the TSH is the initial mechanism regulating your thyroid, but your body has more and more ways besides the TSH of regulating the free hormones. Although the free hormones have a shorter period, they are often the last to show the course adjustments. So if someone was receiving the right amount of thyroid, then their dose started going higher, the TSH would start to drop for a while before the free hormones elevated and because your body would be working hard to eliminate the excess thyroid hormone, you would not have extra levels of hormone.

The first step is the TSH is suppressed and this is where many alternative doctors say, "That's okay. You can keep someone on that dose. You can keep dosing them higher." The partially responsible doctors will say, "At least you can do that until the free hormones elevate." They think that the free hormones are more indicative of your status than the TSH is yet they are not. They are indicative of your body's regulatory mechanisms once the TSH has started to shift. So when you are being dosed and your TSH is being pushed down you are subjected to side effects and complications.

All the side effects and complications are real. Since I see so many patients who were originally treated by other doctors, I have seen every side effect happen. People given too much thyroid hormone can have greater rates of palpitations leading to a stroke through atrial fibrillation, greater risk of dementia, greater risk of osteoporosis, higher rates of muscle tissue wasting leading to overt death, and much higher rates of premature brain aging. These complications are real. Whenever your TSH is pushed below a specific range and a doctor is telling you that it is safe, it is not safe. Again, these are well written in literature but I have also seen them firsthand because I see so many thyroid patients treated by many doctors and many of them come into my practice with this TSH being suppressed and they obviously have complications.

The free hormones will not shift initially when the TSH goes low. Therefore, commonly someone will see that and that will further make them convinced that their efforts to raise the dose are appropriate because they say, "Hey, I raised the dose. At first, I felt better. I was not as tired. I was more energetic. And now my free hormones are low so obviously I need more thyroid" and they keep taking more and more and the free hormones do not catch up. Now eventually they do. A point is reached where your body cannot eliminate thyroid hormone as fast as it is trying to in the face of an overdose, and when that happens the free hormones do elevate finally and they become high. One small caveat if you do measure someone's Free T3 in the first several hours after they take a dose of medication that contains T3 – such as Cytomel or desiccated thyroid – it is always going to be high. That can even happen if they are on a good dose and the TSH is not suppressed – if it is not pushed down too low. However, aside from that, the free hormones only elevate after your body's thyroid elimination mechanisms have been well exhausted. Once that happens then they start to go up.

Generally at that point people have just unmistakable, unavoidable hyperthyroid complications that force them to start tapering down their dosage. The difficult part is that their bodies are just maxed out at how fast they are dumping thyroid hormone so even if a taper is a move in the right direction, it does not feel like it at first. You are receiving too much of it and your body is getting rid of it as fast as it can so when you lower the dose you are still dumping it out fast and you obviously feel more hypothyroid. Therefore, it can be an ordeal to take someone like that at that brink and work back down to healthy dosing. It seems counterintuitive based upon their symptoms and their experience. Before, when they raised the dose they felt better and now we are lowering the dose and they are feeling worse and it seems so obvious that it is the wrong direction. However, commonly when they do come down to a good range they have had their symptoms improve again because now their body has the hormone and it is not dumping it out fast.

So the symptoms of too much thyroid can look like the symptoms of too little thyroid – counterintuitive and difficult for people to grasp – many doctors get it wrong and they overdose patients, subjecting them not only to danger but also not controlling their symptoms. You cannot make someone lose weight or become more energetic by just giving them more and more thyroid because their body is going to dump out the thyroid faster and faster. With dosing, it takes gentle working to move the TSH somewhere close to 1.0 – perhaps slightly below it – and the free hormones should be at a reasonable range.

Now we will talk in a little more detail about fine-tuning of dosage. The free hormones should be at reasonable proportions. They should be roughly midrange and they should be rather proportional to one another. If one is higher, the other should be higher. However, they should be in the range – not on either extreme. If they are different – one is high and one is low – that either means the test was taken after a dose was given or the body is having some bottlenecking. A good conversion is not happening – and we will talk about that.

Now further steps to take into account with fine-tuning would be thyroid antibodies and reverse T3. Thyroid antibodies are a sign and they are a problem. They are both indicators of Hashimoto as Disease but by themselves they also do make dosing more difficult and is the reason for these hormones – these antibodies – attacking proteins within the active hormone. This breaks down your gland. These are proteins involved with reactions inside your gland but they are often proteins embedded within the circulating hormones. So when they are active and circulating they are going to neutralize many of your circulating thyroid hormone, meaning that you will have either symptoms of too little thyroid or your symptoms will be more erratic where sometimes you feel like there is too much and sometimes too little. Therefore, when the thyroglobulin or thyroid peroxidase – the two main antibodies – is greatly elevated, that can be problematic.

Now there are situations when people actually have an overlap between Hashimoto's antibody reactions and Grave's antibody reactions when the thyroid stimulates immunoglobulin antibody. It is worth looking for at least once in someone's case and if it is present, it should be tracked as one more way to help reach ideal levels. With Hashimoto's Disease, you can have that and not be positive for Hashimoto's antibodies. Not unusual, in fact. Upward of 40% of patients with Hashimoto's may not present positive, active, circulating antibodies, and it does take evaluation through ultrasound to obtain a sense of the immune response.

Antibodies should be evaluated, especially when someone is symptomatic and they are somehow not feeling well – whether it is the weight or the hair, the fatigue. If they are greatly up they should be both addressed, not only to slow the disease process but also to manage symptoms, then also to prevent secondary autoimmune diseases from forming. When the antibodies are up that raises the risk of continuing thyroid inflammation and that creates greater risk for the structural problems – the nodules, the goiters and the cancer. Therefore, the antibodies are important to manage.

Now the other factor with them is that the more things you are attacking unnecessarily, the more other things you might start attacking unnecessarily. The more active one autoimmune process – such as Hashimoto's Disease – the greater your risk of having other autoimmune diseases form is – such as Lupus or rheumatoid arthritis or celiac. Therefore, it is good to keep these antibodies under control not only for your symptoms but also for your long-term health and minimizing complications.

So what are the main variables that affect that? Well, a couple of the big ones are other things that affect your immune system and the biggest ones there are going to be infections and allergies. Moreover, infections are commonly things from outside your body but they can also be internal. We talked a little about candida and dysbiosis before and that can be a big factor with this. Any chronic, low-grade infections inside the intestinal tract or the sinuses or the blood – such as Epstein Barr Virus – can drive that elevation in antibodies. Then allergies can also be triggers for that and we did talk about those earlier as well. Anything you are exposed to through the air, your diet, or your skin – that can aggravate your immunity and therefore raise your reaction to other things your body – is inclined to attack.

Another big variable receiving a lot of press lately has been Reverse T3. Many do not need to worry about this but it can be useful in cases that are more complicated.

Some people are diagnosed, and they are placed on a T4 medication. They bring their TSH back to the abysmal normal range – forget the ideal range. Yet they do well. They had their symptoms clear up and they are getting back on with things. More power to them. However, for others it is not that easy. So, the more complicated and involved someone's case is – the more difficult of a time they have had – the more variables it is worth looking at and addressing. I do not always lead with screening for reverse T3 levels, simply because it is not that consistent an indicator and for many people it is not relevant. However, there are those who are dialed in, their TSH is ideal, free hormones are healthy, they are on a good kind of medication, we have their antibodies controlled, but they still may be symptomatic. Then this is often the next step I will take. Moreover, it does apply to some.

Now the shortcoming is a big gap in how to treat it effectively and how to interpret it effectively. The conventional world is none. They do not ever test for this and do not do anything about it so it is not even on their radar map. The alternative world, the most common approach – this was brought into popularity by Doctor Dennis Wilson and he talked about the condition he called "Wilson's Syndrome" – breaking the rules for naming diseases. The normal rule is that if you do discover a brand-new disease process, which arguably he did not, someone else may choose to name that disease process after you – well after you died. However, no one gets to name it after themselves within their lifetime. So anyway, he called this thing Wilson's Syndrome, in which a high amount of reverse T3 is made and he argued that the remedy was to give more T3. Logical enough. It sure makes sense that if we are not receiving enough T3 we can give more T3. However, the problem here is that it does not represent a thorough understanding of how this whole process works.

When reverse T3 is made, it is not because of error and this process lacks real understanding in the alternative medicine world. A condition called Euthyroid Sick Syndrome or Non-Thyroidal Illness has been well recognized to occur with patients who are sick in many ways such as heart disease, kidney disease, major infections, or some malignancy. However, when you are sick your body intentionally makes more Reverse T3 out of your thyroid hormones as an adaptive response. It is an intentional way of slowing your machinery because there are a few loose screws in the machinery.

I think of my father learning how to drive truck on the farm. His dad would put a can of beans under the throttle so he could not step it down as far. This was so he was not in danger of exceeding a speed that he could control. Much the same as what reverse T3 is doing. Your body is intentionally putting a can of beans under the throttle so you cannot overdo it. When you are sick – when something is off somehow – you are tired and you want to take it easy and rest and when it is bad enough your body will actually force the issue. It will block your throttle, so to speak, and force you to further slow, which is what happens.

The Wilson's Syndrome model proposes that reverse T3 blocks your body's formation of healthy T3 and he argues that reverse T3 blocks the T3 receptors in the cell membrane. However, these pathways – these chemical pathways – have been so thoroughly studied and researched that we know in great chemical detail how they work and how they operate, and this proposal is not how they work or how they operate. If there were any way by which reverse T3 blocked T3, then this mechanism would exist in most living creatures that have thyroid hormone, which is most mammals. Therefore, if this mechanism worked in such a willy nilly fashion, we would not have made it out of the ocean.

It happens all the time that we make a bunch of reverse T3 when we are sick and not feeling well, and then we shut it off again. Even with normal health, we make more Reverse T3 than active T3. Therefore, the proposal that reverse T3 blocks T3 is the opposite of the truth. Reverse T3 actually encourages T3. When you receive too much of it, that actually slows the mechanisms and your body then eventually goes back to a state of balance unless some underlying stressor occurs. The solution for reverse T3 is not to give T3 –stomping on the gas pedal when you are not in good control of the truck or when your body is sick and strained somehow. The solution is to figure out "Why is the reverse T3 being formed?"

A number of things that can cause this are beyond the scope and relevance of this book, but suffice to say the solution is to have a good conventional or alternative diagnostician to sort where the stressors may be. In addition, your symptoms often point to that. However, we think about any of your major organs, your body's metabolic processes, your bone marrow functions, and any latent, hidden cancers. Something is off when you are forming a lot of T3 and it should definitely be uncovered. The act of uncovering it and addressing it is the way to remedy the excess reverse T3 formation. The remedy does not come by simply giving more T3. All that does is subjects the person to more of the hyperthyroid side effects and complications.

So a little about things that would prompt a dose change. Imagine a scenario in which we have someone well dialed in. They have their scores right and they are feeling well. This is not to say that the scores and the labs are the be-all and end-all for all symptoms, because they are not but they are a big step. When the scores are not right, it becomes one of the easier addressable opportunities to help someone feel better. It is one of the first steps to regaining full health. So let us say someone's scores are right. There may be things that can be expected to change in their dose needs.

One of those would be other medications and this can mean things taken and acting on the intestinal tract and affecting absorption but it can also mean things taken that affect how your body utilizes thyroid hormones. The list of medications that can skew this is long. What I suggest to someone is that if they are going on a new medicine do consider monitoring their thyroid scores over the following several weeks and months. Most any new medication can skew this. Now you should not be taking anything else with your thyroid. So any new medicine – take it at a separate time.

A difficult thing is how to handle antacids. People are often put on antacid therapy. Ideally, it would not be long term but sometimes it is needed in the short term and the morning is the most effective time for controlling acid reflux during the daytime hours. If you were to do things properly, you would take the thyroid first then wait for about an hour, then take your antacids then wait for about an hour and eat – a big nuisance. I would be afraid the person would not be having a decent breakfast. They are probably going to run out of the door having just taken the pills and even then they are probably not going to do it right often because it is not easy to adhere to this regime.

They have shown that your thyroid dose works just as well if you do take it at nighttime with the consideration that you should have an empty stomach and you should not have just taken a calcium supplement. Therefore, if you are taking an antacid and you do need to, what I would recommend for you is to take your thyroid at nighttime. You can take your calcium at a different time of day with a meal but I would not take it with your thyroid but take your thyroid right before you go to bed. For your overall health, you are going to sleep better and be more apt to break down your fat stores if you are going to bed on an empty stomach anyway. A good policy in general is to go to bed on an empty stomach, or at least several hours after eating. You can take your thyroid right then. They have done many well-designed studies on symptoms and blood levels and it makes no difference. It is a matter of personal preference.

Some people who do not take antacids also choose to do this just for convenience purposes. They may wish to wake, promptly have breakfast, and go on with their day – nothing wrong with that. You can obtain the same benefits and there are no negative issues. Whichever method you keep, you would want to stick with. If you were jumping back and forth that would cause your levels to be somewhat variable. Either method is fine but just be consistent with it.

Now other things that can skew your need for thyroid hormones would be any kind of hormone replacement therapy.

That includes everything from the most well done, bioidentical regime, to a high dose oral contraceptive. So natural or synthetic, both can skew the thyroid. Now in general, progesterone compounds tend to increase your body's utilization of thyroid. There are some cases where someone is only on a progesterone replacement, they may need a little less thyroid. Often, progesterone only has no significant impact. Now the other type of common treatment is estrogen replacement. As a generalization again, estrogen replacement will require someone to need a little more thyroid replacement and you can see the opposite for both so the smartest approach in those cases is closer, more frequent monitoring.

A good rule about monitoring is to check after six weeks when something has happened to affect your levels or caused a big shift in your levels. If you are unchanged from where you were last time, look at it in three months. It is probably going to be fine then. But if it is off – if it has shifted – then check it again short term and check it short term until it comes right – until it is at a healthy range. Once it is healthy then start to back off and there is no real advantage in testing as often. But starting some version of hormone replacement therapy – whether it is subdermal pellets or topical creams or sublingual lozenges or shots or pills – anything like that, it is worth closely screening for thyroid status in the following months.

Along the same lines, pregnancy will also represent the big shift in your body's hormonal balance. When going into pregnancy, it is especially important to closely dial in thyroid status. I would even argue for fertility purposes. The act of becoming pregnant, of course, will not skew your thyroid's needs but you are going to do your best going into pregnancy if you are already dialed in and stable and you are also going to have your best chances of conceiving and surviving that first trimester with a healthy baby. So if you are planning pregnancy, it is a good time to become dialed in, get your dosages right and once you become pregnant check it rather frequently. Again, the more stable it is, the longer you can go. Never go more than two and a half months or three months at the most between testing when you are pregnant. If it is varying – if it is fluctuating – then you should be testing it between four and six weeks.

The most common scenario is that pregnant women need a little more of a higher dose than they do in the non-pregnant state, then correspondingly, they will most commonly need to decrease after the pregnancy. However, immune changes in pregnancy can do the opposite and actually require lower dosages rather than higher dosages. It does take good, regular testing for the health of Mom and the health of the baby, then afterward things may be going back to where they were prior but they could be resetting in other ways too.

Other big shifts would be the starting and the ending of menstrual cycles. So if a girl has already been diagnosed as having thyroid disease when her menstrual cycles start – age 11 to 13 nowadays is more common – then that alone could shift a need in her replacement. Then also going through perimenopause and menopause – those fluctuations and those winding down of hormones often do signal needed changes as well. Perimenopause – there can be many times when a pattern we call "estrogen dominance" emerges, meaning that the amount of estrogen relative to progesterone has increased and that can be from just high estrogen or from low progesterone or from both of those. Any of those scenarios that involve estrogen dominance can commonly make the woman require a higher dose of thyroid treatment. Then the menopausal process of a woman who is not undergoing replacement therapy – she is going to have less active estrogen after menopause has set in so she may need a smaller dose. So generally more during perimenopause, less during menopause. If hormone replacement is being used, then that is different.

Another variable that can make someone's thyroid dose change is a big change in body weight. The dose that you need is a function of your chemistry, how much you are making by yourself but also it is a function of just how much body mass you have that needs thyroid hormone. So if your amount of body mass goes down by 20% because you did an awesome job on your dieting and your hormones were dialed in well – cool – but you are likely to need about 20% less thyroid hormone because of that and the opposite is also true. If you were to go up by 5 or 10% for various reasons, you have mass that needs thyroid hormone now so your dose should be expected to be increased to compensate for that.

Then the last thing that can cause dosing changes rather commonly would be seasonal shifts and this is less a factor than it could be because we are well climate controlled. Most of us are indoors often in our lives. However, I definitely see people who need higher dosages in the winter and lower dosages in the summer. It is not unusual and can occur so you need to be aware of that. For many people it is enough if their blood levels shift slightly but they will not need a prompting of a change of dose.

Some people do need different amounts at various times of the year. Tt can become rather predictable if they are well regulated and we can just plan for it. This is truer if you are in an extreme climate that has a bigger variation in temperatures from one season to the next. So generally, colder climates – people need more thyroid and warmer climates – they need a little less. So be aware of that. This can also happen if someone is moving from one part of the country to another that has a different climate. Seasons and external temperature can also shape what someone needs with their thyroid dosing.

Chapter Summary

Thyroid medicines are categorized as natural and synthetic. Natural hormones are derived from porcine (pig) sources and contain the 3 main human thyroid hormones. Natural thyroid may be more helpful for those with Hashimoto's. The goal of treatment is the correction of symptoms. Symptoms should not be ignored. However, basing a thyroid dose solely on symptoms will not give the best outcomes. This is because symptoms can be the same on too much or too little thyroid. Some doctors ignore lab values completely saying they treat patients not lab values. Yet to treat patients well and really help their symptoms in the long term, we cannot ignore lab values. With many other conditions like diabetes or high blood pressure, it is also known that symptoms are not accurate reflections of the condition.

Action Steps

6. If you are not feeling your best on levothyroxine therapy, consider Natural Desiccated Thyroid.

7. Have your dose adjusted to target a TSH of close to or just below 1.0.

8. If TSH is good and free T3, free T4 or reverse T3 are not, look for allergies, infections, toxins or lacking nutrients.

Chapter 4

Losing Weight

Chapter At a Glance

- Too much thyroid does not help body weight

- Thyroid effects basal metabolic rate - this is a larger source of calorie loss than exercise.

- Weight loss by the numbers

- Thyroid disease links to diabetes and liver disease

- Best types of exercise

- Ideal macronutrient ratios

- Adjusting meal frequency

- Value of food logs

What in the world can I eat and how can I lose weight? I put these together because in so many cases they do overlap. Of course, the diet is a big part of achieving ideal body weight. Aside from body weight, there are some particular concerns about which foods are or are not compatible for those who have Hashimoto's. Some concerns are real and some are not.

One of the most pressing issues we hear repeatedly is how can you hit an ideal body weight. For many people, this is a big dilemma. This does not affect everyone with thyroid disease but it does affect many. It actually can affect those who have mild hyperthyroidism just as much as it can affect those who have hypothyroidism. Often doctors or patients think if they would take higher doses of thyroid, it will make things easier for losing weight. This is actually not true. The lack of thyroid can cause weight gain, but a tolerable excess of thyroid does not consistently cause weight loss.

There does come a point where if the excess is large enough, eventually wasting does occur. This is not healthful, sustainable fat loss. It is severe anxiety, cardiac damage, and loss of muscle and bone.

One of the most troubling examples of this was Kent. He had a diagnosis of Graves' disease but was unwilling to undergo treatment for it. He believed if he were somewhat "hyper", it would give him more energy and make it easier to maintain his weight. I tried so hard to educate him about the real dangers he was risking but I did not do a good enough job at it. Every few years he would come in to see me when he was feeling especially awful. He would go on natural thyroid blockers but only take small amounts for brief periods.

One year, Kent came to see me with concerns about recent onset swelling of his feet. It was severe. His ankles had at least tripled in diameter. The swelling was so extensive there was fluid draining through his skin. He also mentioned a troubling dry cough had come around the same time. Ignorance would have been bliss for me in this situation. Unfortunately, the second I saw his feet I already suspected late stage congestive heart failure. The cough just confirmed it. He was also having a fluid build-up in his lungs. I knew that with aggressive care under a skilled cardiologist, he could buy a little more time, but not much. I also doubted whether he would follow up with a cardiologist. He did not. A few weeks later, I received a call from the county medical examiner. Kent was found dead in his apartment. My name was found in his paperwork, and I was the only medical contact they could find. Extra thyroid can kill.

The problem is whenever your intake of thyroid medications is above what your body's needs are, you will dump out the excess hormone, and it simply does not result in making you burn more calories. It can actually do the opposite often.

So the problem though is with thyroid disease, there is often too little thyroid hormone to encourage the burning of fuel. The body therefore stores more fuel.

Now our body weight really is a function of calories in versus calories out. Body fat is not so simple and we will talk about that further. However, our output of calories, as opposed to our input of calories, primarily governs our weight. The output of calories has two primary sources – the passive output and the active output. When we think about burning calories, we think about the active output. This is when you are out exercising, playing, or doing any type of physical work.

I think about the body as like a car that cannot shut off. It always at least stays in idle mode. The active calories are how many miles you are going to drive the car. That is how much gas you are going to burn. However, the passive calories – that is the car idling continuously. Even if you are not on a trip the body – as a car – is always running so you are burning fuel continuously. For many of us the passive calories – the idling calories – result in a much larger number than the active calories. We frankly burn much more calories throughout the day total resting than we do during active prescribed bouts of exercise. We call these passive calories our resting metabolic rate.

In numbers, most women are burning between about 1,400 and 2,000 calories per day passively, then whatever extra they might do from exercise. The number of calories we burn from exercise is always less than we think. There are many charts, graphs, heart rate monitors, and devices at the gym saying, "Here is how many calories you burned" and usually they are not accurate. I will give you guys a quick background. I have done many different hobbies in the past. One of which was I spent a few years as a competitive cyclist. Cyclists burn many calories from long rides – 100-mile rides – and we had to refuel properly. We had to replace those calories to be ready for the next ride. If we did not get enough food we were simply too weak to ride again. However, if we have too much we would gain weight. Weight gain could be counterproductive for our speed on a bike.

I am unlucky in that I could easily gain if I rode that much and just eat what I wanted. I had to really count the calories and estimate how many I burned. There were many ways to measure how many I had burned. These included my bike computer, my heart rate monitor to charts and graphs to the online calorie counters. Yet when I actually ate that many calories, I gained weight quickly.

At some point in my training I used a device called the Power Meter, which shows your actual output of power in watts. There are some easy conversions between watts and calories. Once I saw a measured power output as opposed to an estimated caloric output I saw all the other ways I was estimating calories were overgenerous. Often by a factor of twofold. So if you see a chart that says you burned this many calories while you were doing an aerobics class for an hour, the real number is probably close to half.

A calorie output with exercise is much smaller than the calories we burn from resting metabolism. The big issue with thyroid disease is that the resting metabolism is suppressed. I have seen several numbers but some as high as 50%. This means your body will only burn half the calories at rest it would otherwise do if you did not have thyroid disease, making things difficult to manage the body weight. Our diet – we have to consume at least about 1,200 calories per day just to meet our basic nutritional needs in protein and healthy fats and essential nutrients. If we are having to go much less than that, we are going to be losing our lean mass and becoming malnourished and unhealthy. With thyroid disease all too often, the resting metabolism is below that range.

If you are someone who has really struggled with the weight, an intelligent thing to do is have that measured. There is a device called a ReeVue or an indirect calorimeter and they are readily available. A good many gyms, trainers, nutritionists, doctors do have these devices and they can do easy tests to accurately show what your resting metabolism is. For those who have thyroid disease it might be lower than you would expect and it is handy to know because if it is below a particular range then weight loss is more about correcting thyroid function than it is about achieving a caloric deficit.

The numbers for weight loss of calories are that it takes about 3,500 calories to equal a pound of body weight. If we ever have a deficit that large, we are going to lose about a pound of weight. About a 500 deficit per day for a week gives you roughly 3,500 calories, which would require about a pound of weight per week. Now if your metabolism is slow you have to be eating as little as 700-600 calories to achieve that, which is not safe, nor is it healthy.

With body weight, one of the first steps is getting the thyroid dose correct and we did talk about that at length in the last section. You need to be sure you get your TSH close to 1 – perhaps slightly below it but not too much below it. You need to be on the right amount of thyroid replacement and the right type of thyroid replacement. Often this is one of the benefits people see when they switch from a T4-only medicine, such as Synthroid or levothyroxine, to desiccated thyroid, probably because of the T3 and T2 we talked of in the last chapter. But if your weight has been a struggle and you are on a T4-only medication I would prioritize the change as one of your first steps before you beat yourself up too hard about trying much of anything else because some cases can make it go much easier.

I have talked briefly about weight versus fat – we always talk about weight loss – but what we really want is long-term fat loss. These are different. The calories issue is important but it is not all of it. With a group of people, you could put them all on the same number of calories and they will not all get the same outcome. There will be an average response but there are many who will have persistent weight gain even though they are at a low enough calorie range. People are different in that way. We really want to achieve fat loss and we need to dial in our body's chemistries.

Therefore, the first step is really to achieve the right amounts of thyroid. Another thing to look at if you have had a difficult time and you have a lower metabolism is cortisol and we will talk more about that in future topics but high cortisol will work against your body's weight loss efforts. This is especially the case if someone is taking prednisone or other types of oral cortisol analogs to help manage inflammation. It is almost impossible to lose weight in that situation. Then some people just make too much by themselves continuously.

A big factor too, along the same lines, is insulin. People become numb to insulin. Now the role of insulin is to become burned. If it cannot get inside the cell, it cannot burn properly and insulin is what brings it in. Now the problem is we are exposed to more and more starch – especially processed starch – than we ever were in our distant past and at some point it requires more and more insulin for us to process the same amount of starch and we call that "insulin resistance." If we have to make plenty of insulin, we are more likely to be in a state of storage than we are of burning and we are going to have a difficult time burning starch for fuel. Therefore, if there are concerns about insulin resistance it can take more of an aggressive lower carbohydrate approach. You would not want to go to none but reductions can make a considerable difference and we will talk more about macronutrient ratios too.

Insulin resistance can be directly measured, and accurate insulin tests for morning fasting can be helpful. It can also be indirectly determined. If someone is prone to having blood sugar imbalances – and people really know this – it is often not apparent on single fasting blood tests. However, people know whether they have blood sugar problems if they really feel awful, if they are late for a meal, or if they have a sugary snack and nothing else for a while they are going to crash, feel dizzy, weak, and emotionally unstable. That alone points towards some insulin resistance. Strong tendencies towards midbody weight gain – so a higher waist circumference, greater than hips perhaps – can also be factors of there being more insulin resistance. Then those who have had high levels of triglycerides or low levels of HDL cholesterol likely have some degree of insulin resistance. If so, it will take some management and we will talk about macronutrients. Lipoic acid can be of benefit. Adding cinnamon to the diet in rather large amounts can also be of benefit.

Then regular, higher intensity type exercise can help. What we call the "chronic cardio" or the long, slow, gentle type cardio training may not be as helpful. It probably does take briefer bursts of higher intensity exercise to achieve the good benefits of reversing the insulin resistance. Thankfully, that is easier on the time schedule as it takes less time to achieve. There are good high-intensity interval training workouts you can do within twenty minutes. With less than thirty minutes you can have a phenomenal workout that gives you good metabolic changes not only for insulin resistance but also for cardiovascular wellness, as well as "post-exercise burn," meaning it can leave your body in a state of heightened calorie burning for a good time so is excellent, time efficient, and more effective in general.

A big thing now is just having calories appropriate but if someone has a slow metabolism the next thing to look at is going to be the macronutrients and the ratios of protein, fat, and starch, which can be huge. This is such an important factor. Our diet receives calories from three sources and is protein, fat, or carbohydrate – also called starch. You could also carbohydrate sugar and the term "sugar" is used in two ways. To a nutritionist or biochemist, sugar often means all carbohydrate but when we are talking in more common terms sugar tends to mean the simple processed form of carbohydrate. We receive calories from three sources and it is important how those particular sources relate to one another. Ideally, we would receive good but appropriate amounts of all of them with each of our meals. This is something to where it does not really balance throughout the day and this is somewhat intuitive. You really would not do well if you had just a meal of chicken breasts, then just a meal of popcorn, then just a meal of butter. That would not give you healthy, steady energy levels and it would not leave you satisfied either – maybe the butter meal but not the others.

Therefore, you really want a good ratio with each of your meals. Your blood sugar – the more it has to fluctuate, the more your body is likely to move into the storage mode and out of the burning mode. The biggest variable is those ratios but especially those ratios for your first several meals. Each time you eat determines your body's hormonal balance for the next 6 to 12 hours. Your first few meals have the biggest impact on the day whether you are able to burn calories or store calories. So one of the most common issues I see as an obstacle for people is just not having enough protein for breakfast. If there is too little protein for your first meal, your body's metabolism will slow for the whole day as a result and you will find yourself more hungry and more in a storage state.

I had a patient many years back who had thyroid disease and weight loss resistance, and that was the whole linchpin for her. We saw Anne – we can call her Anne – she was fatigued as well and she was at appropriate thyroid levels. She had no big issues with other hormones. Cortisol was well regulated. Insulin and estrogen were reasonable. However, she was fatigued and she could not lose weight. Often these things go hand in hand. It seems counterintuitive but what is happening is the body cannot properly burn fuel, you are storing fuel, you are not getting the energy, and you are not breaking down the fat stores at the same time. The same thing causing the fatigue is the direct thing causing the resistant weight.

Therefore, in Anne's case, it turned out she was eating healthful, unprocessed foods, most of which were made at home. Some were even grown at home. They had their own garden. However, the diet was heavy in grains and vegetables only, especially the first several meals, which actually were more grains and fruits, and those are not uncommon. Many people will cut out dairy and some will cut out eggs with concerns about allergenicity, then they tend to focus on mostly just grains and sometimes fruit or vegetables. Certainly, those foods have their place and are especially healthy, but if there are no dense sources of protein then we do not really have the stimulation for our metabolic fires.

So often people think, "Well if I just have beans or nuts and seeds or cheese, I'll get enough protein." The problem is those foods do contain protein but they do not primarily contain protein. Beans and legumes are wonderful foods. They are my favorite version of carbohydrate. They are the slowest metabolized by the body and they are the richest in fiber and nutrients. However, their principal contribution is carbohydrate so they are higher in protein than grains are but they are nowhere near the protein content of poultry, for example. They are primarily giving your body more carbohydrates. They are good carbs but they are not a predominantly protein food, then nuts and seeds and cheeses – they are primarily fat contributors.

Therefore, without dense protein with your first few meals, you will have a suppressed metabolism. In Anne's case, we saw that change. We added some protein to the breakfast with salmon, most commonly, and some protein powders. Without really changing her caloric intake her energy levels went back to where they should have been, which allowed her to exercise. Even before the exercise kicked in, she noticed the pounds coming off, especially around the midsection. Her response was typical. The initial intake of protein really sets the whole stage for how the day's metabolism will work.

Therefore, in numbers, the good ratios to get are going to be roughly a third or fewer calories from protein – 25-30%, about the same amount for fat – 25-30% and the balance from carbohydrate. This is an easy thing to know whether you are doing diet logging. We will talk a little more about that. It is a helpful tool – kind of like training wheels, especially at first. Once you get the hang of it and figure out how to balance well you can ditch training wheels and still ride pretty good. Same way with food logging – once you figure out what are the right ratios, what are the right calorie intakes for yourself, you do not have to log continuously. It can be certainly tedious at some point. So yeah, a big first step is getting the macronutrients – the ratios – right.

Then the next one is figuring out the actual servings for these foods and the number of meals. There is no magic formula that is true for everyone on how many times we have to eat throughout the day. There has been much data lately suggesting meals should be more frequent and, there certainly are those who do prefer that and probably feel better for it. I am one of those. However, a blanket statement is not necessary for everyone. Many people can do well on fewer meals – two –

throughout the day. It really does come down to the total number of calories, then also the ratio of the protein and fat and the starch. Those two variables are much more important than the number of meals.

So figure out the number of meals that works best for your blood sugar, your convenience – your lifestyle – the meals all do take some time. It is convenient to eat less frequently. Figure out the number that works best for you, and then stick with that. Then make a line in the sand that this is your frequency for eating is X-number of meals throughout the day. Whether that is two, three, or four or for some five – then be consistent about not exceeding that number. If you are not engaged in one of the designated mealtimes then just do not eat. Just leave it until later. Also, get a sense on just eyeballing portion sizes of the protein, fat, and starch to have in your meals. Those two steps can go a long way toward achieving weight without there being detailed counting or detailed steps. If you find yourself at a proper number of meals and a good average serving size and your weight is not moving then slightly decrease the serving size.

Here is a good starting place. If you are doing some regular physical activity, you can do fine with some healthful starches in the diet. You can go too low in those, which can actually be counterproductive. You would want to get roughly one-half of a cup of a dense carbohydrate per meal if you are doing some physical exercise. By healthful dense carbohydrate, I would include beans of all types – pinto, navy, northern, garbanzos, you name it; they are wonderful foods – or you could choose whole grain brown rice, some cooked sweet potato, or some steel cut oats if this were a morning meal but about half a cup in volume of some dense healthful carbohydrate. About what you could easily put in one hand without it overflowing – not a large amount. The idea of the plate spilling with pasta and a small meatball on top is not the right kind of ratio. Think of carbohydrates more of as a garnish.

Therefore, the meal then should also have roughly the same amount of volume of dense protein so about half a cup or slightly more of meat, fish, poultry, eggs, or cottage cheese – if you are not reacting to them. This can also be protein powders for a variety of purposes but you would want that to be roughly the same volume as your carbohydrate.

Then the remaining amount of your meal, you are welcome to fill totally with all kinds of non-starchy vegetables, including almost anything you would commonly see in a salad or a stir-fry. This is going to be lettuce, onions, broccoli, cauliflower, and greens. I would put carrots in this list too. Tomatoes, bell peppers – you name it – any fruit or vegetable except sweet potatoes, potatoes, or corn. Things like beets and carrots – they certainly do have some carbohydrate but the amount you get in each serving is so small that it is negligible. No one has ever gained weight from binging on carrots or beets. You do want to monitor the denser versions of starch so watch the corn and the potatoes. They are more powerful. As for the other vegetables – eat them freely. Eat them to give yourself good satiety and let yourself fill up on them. Our sense of being full is more tightly coupled to our volume of food than it is to our caloric intake of food.

A good meal is going to be about half a cup to a cup of a dense protein, about half a cup of a dense carbohydrate, then the remaining number of fruits and vegetables. If you are not doing much regular exercise, if you are not on a particular day, or if you are more weight loss resistant you can safely diminish the carbohydrate. I would not go much lower than one to two quarter-cup servings throughout the day. What happens is when we consume a little carbohydrate we actually make carbohydrate by ourselves? That is fine but if we go too low, we actually result in making more than we would if we would have just eaten a little. We could actually make internally more starch than is desirable. You do not want to go down to zero versions of carbohydrate. You want some healthful starch with your meals – not much less than about a quarter cup a few times per day.

Remember the number of meals is not critical. Do not feel you have to eat five or six times a day if it is a nuisance for you and not enjoyable. Find the number that works for you and stick with that. If you do find yourself hungry outside a mealtime and desperate to snack then any non-starchy produce can be fair game. The caloric impact those foods have is minimal.

Here are a few good, simple rules. Do not consume calories from liquids. People ask me about "Well, what's better – soy milk or rice milk or almond milk?" and we will talk about particular foods but overall water-milk is the best. We really do not need milk when we are not babies. The idea of taking in liquid calories – that only comes up among mammals when they are growing fast. It does not really come up for adult mammals at all in the natural world. Liquid calories – they enter our bodies so quickly we have no choice but to store them. We really cannot burn them as quickly as we receive them so in general liquid calories become the low hanging piece of fruit easy to cut out. Many papers have shown that when someone has had issues with their weight, just by taking soda out of the diet (if they have not already) can be a factor of 12 to 16 pounds per year on average – of fat. It is hugely powerful, and if you are taking in liquid calories then this is your first step.

Now if you need a little dash of some creamer in your coffee or tea – dairy or non-dairy– I would not worry too much about it. Keep it down to a tablespoon or so, and minimize the addition of liquid to cereals. Overall, it is not a meal with good nutrient ratios – it is going to be starch and sugary starch on starch. Nowadays, some better-quality protein powders do not have carbohydrate – they can be mixed with water and work well as a topping on cereal or oatmeal. It is a useful complement too, as you are getting the starch, the oatmeal, or the cereal as well as the protein with it to give yourself the proper ratios. An easy trick, so just drop any types of drinks with calories – juices, milk, sodas, any sweetened drinks – just avoid those.

The question often comes up about artificially sweetened items – they do not have calories but they are still sweet. Maybe it is a way to get you off the soda or off the juice, but it is a step in the right direction. Some purists argue that "Well, the sweet taste still may cause you to have sweet cravings. It still may affect your metabolism". I have read several studies about this phenomenon but they have not been consistent. Some studies have shown that perhaps sweet things without calories do have a slight effect on us, while other studies have shown that there is no effect. The conclusion I can draw from these conflicting studies is that if these things do affect us it is not in a profoundly negative way – at worst, they are mildly negative.

I personally do not use them regularly but if someone is finding them as an easy way to get off juice or soda, that is splendid. It is a big step in the right direction. Do not beat yourself up. A common thing I will see is something I call "the perfect is the enemy of the good." We can have all these lofty rules and goals and someone might think, "Well if I cannot have organic broccoli that I harvested from my own perfect garden this morning then I am going to eat ice cream", which is probably not the most rational approach. So do not let the perfect be the enemy of the good. If sweetened, non-caloric drinks are something you could use as a step off soda then go for it. If you like water and you do well with it, then it is the best drink. Focus on that, by all means.

Another easy one is that you have the number of meals chosen, planned, know that and keep tabs, then when you have covered your number of meals, the day is done. Know the portions you are going to target per meal. Another good rule of thumb is with the fats – any fats we have in the foods. They find their way in. You do want fish regularly, somewhere around a quarter cup throughout the day of nuts and seeds is healthy as well and aside from that we do not really need to add fats. So for each meal the rule of thumb is that the last joint in your thumb that has a little more than your thumbnail – that is about the volume of oil you would want for any meal. Then if you imagine the rest of your thumb – the volume of that, which is about a tablespoon – that is about the volume you would want of less dense fat like peanut butter or almond butter or a dressing. That is the most you would want per meal total fat from all sources. That is a rule of thumb for fats throughout the meal.

With rates of weight loss – what is realistic, what can happen? It is a good thing to know about, both for proper expectations but also for knowing when you are on the right rate. You should not be seeing that your weight is reducing at a rate that is faster than about half a pound – maybe a pound – a week aside from the first few weeks. The first few weeks it can go quicker then after that if it is more than half a pound or a pound a week it is probably not going to last and you are probably losing more muscle mass. So ideal rates of weight loss are about half a pound to a pound per week, and this is one of those things where slow and steady wins the race. If it is much faster than that, they have shown from so many big studies that people just universally do regain and it rarely takes more than six months. The most you can maintain on an aggressive diet plan is six months and it is predictable that after that period, people will regress and they are going to regain. The vast majority will finish heavier than they were when they started. You do not want that to happen. You do not want the yo-yo dieting. Those problems alone are greater than just the weight. Slow and steady is what is appropriate, which is useful too because at a rate that gentle, you can maintain your activity and still feel well and not be obsessing about foods.

A helpful thing for getting the numbers right is using food logs and I am a fan of these. I personally use one these days called My Fitness Pal. I used one called My Food Diary for years in the past. They are both extremely handy. There is also one called Calorie King. There are probably some newer competitors in the market nowadays too. The general format with one of these logs is that they will have an online web portal in to which you can log. They often have mobile versions as well, which may be a mobile version of the site or an actual dedicated app for an iPhone or Android that you can use. I like My Fitness Pal these days because it has a barcode scanner and even so many healthful foods – they have barcodes – so rather than going through the process of entering a food and looking it up, you can just scan the barcode of your phone and it will pull up the food accurately most of the time, then just clarify the quantity – if you had all of that or half a serving – however much you had.

Just make sure you have the quantity correct and that it is entered. It is so quick and easy. I like some reporting better on My Food Diary. It has slightly more detailed reports, a little better data organization in my perspective. It is a fee site. It is I think $7 or $9 per month and it does not have the barcode – at least not when I last used it. My Fitness Pal – I like it. It is free. It has the barcode scanner. It has a thorough database of food – it is probably the most extensive – and yeah, it is effective. There are a few useful options.

In addition, the advantage of those things is that they can really teach you about your caloric balance. It can be surprising how quickly calories can add up. The counters can also really teach you about your ratios of protein, fat, and starch. They can give reports to where per meal or per day you can see where your ratios fall. You would not intuitively know that otherwise and once you have the hang of it you do not have to track continuously. One that rather surprised me has been just your intake of fiber and sugar and salt. Those are three really big nutrients that we want to be aware of how much we get and we are often not and we really would not know how much we are being exposed to throughout the day without tracking with some method. Fiber – you want at least 40 grams. Sugar – ideally, you would say less than about 40 grams as a rather aggressive target if you were trying to lose weight.

Then salt – ideally fewer than 2,500 milligrams – and this is huge. Whenever someone has weight issues, which of course, are more common with thyroid disease, there is a greater risk of blood pressure problems and salt does relate to that. The CDC said a few years ago that if we could just take our national salt intake down by one teaspoon per day that could save 90,000 lives per year. Therefore, salt equals stroke and it is a huge correlation. It is something where, for so much of our lives, our bodies can adjust and rid ourselves of the extra salt and it will not affect us. However, at some point we can no longer do this, then we start getting elevations in our blood pressure, and we run the risk of a stroke elevating so a huge factor. It is a fun thing to track our food for a little while, if for nothing else than to know about the salt intake as well as the fiber and the sugar.

Chapter Summary

Weight loss is tough in the best of circumstances. Thyroid disease makes it harder. It is possible and good strategies help. Weight loss also helps your blood sugar and liver function. Exercise is important. Most estimates say it contributes to about 20% of weight loss success. Diet is 80%. Don't think you can exercise your way out of a bad diet.

Action Steps

9. Get your thyroid dose right - this is the easiest way to help your metabolism

10. Consider measurement of your basal metabolic rate to have an accurate calorie target.

11. Eat ⅓ of food volume from quality protein such as fish, poultry, lean meat, cottage cheese, eggs, Greek yogurt or protein powder. This is the best way to stay muscular as you lose weight

12. Try a food log for your first few weeks to get the hang of a healthy calorie target. The more accurately you log, the better the scale will respond. Weight and measure your food to get the hang of it.

Chapter 5

Best and Worst Foods

Chapter At a Glance

- Gluten and thyroid - important for some but not all

- Food intolerances

- Iodine - the Goldilocks mineral - you don't want too much or too little

- Goitrogens - not all created equally, cruciferous veggies and soy

- Digestive flora

Weight loss and what to eat. A question that comes up often is the relevance of being gluten-free for those who have thyroid disease. There has been plenty of awareness about this over the recent past and it has helped but it has also been the source of unnecessary stress for some.

Much data has linked higher rates of celiac disease autoimmune thyroid disease. Both are categorized as autoimmune diseases. This means they are disorders in which the immunity attacks things belonging in the body. For Hashimoto's thyroiditis, these proteins allow the thyroid to form hormones. For celiac disease, these proteins allow the breakdown of the constituents of wheat.

With autoimmune disease in general, if you have one type of it, you have a greater chance of having other types. Therefore, it is no surprise to us there is a higher rate of celiac for those who have Hashimoto's. There has been much data saying that if someone does have celiac disease, which is a more aggressive immune reaction against wheat proteins, there will be a greater rate of damage to the thyroid, then just greater complications in general.

Now some have extrapolated the correlation with celiac disease to argue that everyone who has thyroid disease has to avoid wheat. There is certainly no danger from being off wheat. There is nothing essential we get only from it in our diets and at the same time, there certainly are many negative things about our diets being too high in carbohydrates, especially processed carbohydrates and for the typical American much of that comes from wheat. So on one hand, almost anyone with or without thyroid disease could improve their health by decreasing their intake of processed carbohydrates.

However, do people with thyroid disease have a special reaction to gluten if they do not have celiac? There is no data saying this. Those who have pushed with the wheat connection have cited many studies about wheat as a factor. However, when they back up their claims with studies, all the research they point to is on celiac disease.

If you do not have celiac are not wheat intolerant as such, there is no special danger. There is a real type of gluten intolerance more common than celiac disease. This can affect digestion and overall health in many ways. However, non-celiac gluten intolerance does not affect the immune reactions against the thyroid.

Even so – again, we are often better off having less of our calories from carbohydrates and grains than many of us already get. The principal message is it is intelligent for wheat issues to have testing done for celiac and testing done for gluten intolerance and I will talk about that.

Celiac can be looked for in a several different ways, the most practical is by blood markers and they have now become accurate. In the past, they were less reliable but now any doctor can order a celiac antibody panel from any laboratory, and they can give good data on whether you have tendencies towards celiac disease. The gold standard still is intestinal biopsy. This is done during an upper endoscopy study. A doctor can take a small sample of the villi – the upper part of the small intestinal tract – and by looking at those cells under a microscope, they can say definitively whether there are celiac reactions.

Now a shortcoming about both of those tests is they are not accurate if the person has been avoiding wheat for several months. Perfect avoidance is difficult but some can pull that off. If you have been off wheat for some time and you are tested for celiac, the data may not be conclusive. It may not be accurate. Some would argue the best thing is to go out of our way to eat a fair amount of it in the weeks before testing. The other level of testing is for the gluten intolerance and is more of an IgG – an IgG 4 specifically – type reaction. There has been data saying Hashimoto's is strongly driven by IgG 4 factors, so many types of foods can cause these IgG 4 reactions, and wheat is a more common one. The difference is with this reaction, we would not expect there to be damage to the intestines or damage to the thyroid but there can still be immune complications and worsening of symptoms. Now these reactions are more common than celiac.

The rate of celiac in the general population is somewhere just below 1%. It is higher in some ethnicities than others, but overall less than 1% of the population has overt celiac. When we say it is higher with those who have thyroid disease, it is higher but it is still not everyone. The studies have ranged anywhere from about 3% to about 7% where those having thyroid disease will have celiac. It is not everyone but some, and it is good to know about it if you are in that group. If you are and you are eating wheat regularly, it is difficult on your system. You may not have obvious short-term symptoms but there will be complications over time. There will be nutrients you absorb as effectively. There will be problems with the intestinal apparatus and there can be immune changes as well so it is important.

In addition, I do encourage good screening for general food reactions. Wheat is common, but the most common are dairy and eggs. They are rather typical, and from there on, we can see almost any food reactive for one person here or there. You may have a common reaction like one of those three or it could be something altogether different. The better labs do check for that. It is kind of difficult to notice the more delayed intolerances by trial and error, meaning you could not necessarily peg which food makes you feel bad based upon day-to-day symptoms.

There certainly are times where you can notice that some foods will affect you but sometimes the symptoms come at different times – not so much just after you have eaten the offending food. It can take as much as a week and a half to have symptoms come on after you are eating a reactive IgG type food. Therefore, it is difficult to notice by trial and error in symptoms. However, the blood tests are good nowadays and there are a couple labs I like. I am not financially tied to them. My favorites include US Biotech and Meridian Valley Labs. They are both cost-effective, they have good graphic reports that make sense of things visually and most important, they are accurate.

Many have written about shortcomings with these tests because some labs are not accurate. I would not disagree with that. Over the years, an easy way I could scrutinize these laboratories is by sending them several samples of the same patient's blood on separate occasions. What should happen is that if we have a tube of your blood and another tube of your blood that happens to say "Jane Doe" on it – assuming that is not your name – now they should receive the same report, right? We should get identical reports back. However, that does not happen often. We call that "split sample testing" and it is an easy way to see how accurate the labs are. The two I mentioned have done well on repeated split sample tests, meaning I cannot trip them up – they are accurate.

Now a couple things can happen – there are people who have many things come back reactive. This is typically not representative of long-term reactions. It is typically more representative about their intestinal tract being in an inflamed or irritated state. The reactions are real but they are not reactions we would expect to go on long term.

In a better case scenario, the person can avoid the reactive foods – the worst ones especially – and over time, many of those can diminish. A common thing we can do is to get someone off the worst, most reactive foods, and take things to repair the intestinal lining. Glutamine and n-acetyl glucosamine work well for this. There is a blend called Perma-Clear of these I especially like and see work well. You can then retest 6 or 12 months later, and typically what will happen is many reactions will calm and a few will persist. Those that persist are likely long-term reactions. They are unlikely to change – good or bad. However, the ones that diminished you know were more elevated because the gut was irritated. This is common if you are eating plenty of foods to which you are reactive. You could be eating many things that are culprits for you. That alone can actually bother the gut in ways to makes new reactions. So we call those the functional intolerances as opposed to the long-term intolerances.

The other scenario is that some may have reactions and they may even have symptoms. However, for various reasons their immune systems do not register well in the test tube so it looks like all the foods are nonreactive for them. That is about 5% of the population. Most people seeming to have some symptoms or have a likelihood of having food allergies will have a couple things showing they are better off avoiding long term. They are aware these foods are not their friends and they are better off by avoiding them. There can be a range too. We can see some foods show up highly reactive, in which case we advise thorough avoidance and there can also be foods that are lower or with more moderate levels of reactivity, and then we can encourage something like even a rotation schedule. This can be as simple as not eating a moderately reactive food daily. It can be on a continuum, not just an all-or-nothing reaction.

However, gluten is a common reactive food and the milder intolerances as opposed to celiac are thought to affect perhaps 20% of the population. This is not everyone, but this is some. If you suspect this maybe you, it is worth avoiding it completely for 1 month to see if symptoms improve. There are no dangers to avoiding gluten. Nevertheless, if you have thyroid disease it is also intelligent to be tested to see if there are factors aside from just your day-to-day symptoms that would make it important to avoid.

Now the other important question we hear often is all about iodine. How much iodine do you need? Should I take mega doses of it? Is it dangerous to me? Overall, if you have thyroid disease the principal thing to think about with iodine is avoiding. There is not benefit to adding it. Now you will hear many statements to the contrary and I have been exposed to the fad use of iodine – it is popular now – from patients of mine like many things.

I have seen one patient for many years, and he is a healthy man. Where I practice many people come and go and they are here through the milder times of the year and they are intelligent enough to get out of town when it is hot in the summer and this man is like that. What happens with the care of these people – we call them the "snowbirds" – is I often reassess them as they come back down, then just look at where they are at and what has shifted in their health. I saw this man – someone I enjoy seeing – come back down after the summer, updated his tests and followed up with him. Lo and behold, he had thyroid disease that was not there before, and we found he had a less common type called toxic nodular goiter after we had done a rather thorough evaluation. I asked him about symptoms and it turns out he was getting some symptoms from that, so I asked him about what had gone on before then.

This particular disease is rarer and we generally see it after someone has had rather high dose exposure to iodine. This is most common in imaging studies. Whenever a CT or an MRI is done for whatever reason, they often will use iodine as a contrast. It is used less and less because so many have become aware it is toxic, even in this use. First, I asked him whether he had recently had a CT. He had not. I asked him further and he told me about a new supplement he had been taking called Iodoral. He was told to take it because he had been diagnosed as iodine deficient.

There is a test that has been popularized, called an iodine challenge test. The rationale is someone takes a dose of iodine, and then afterward a urine collection is done. The thought process is that because iodine is passed through the urine, if you need it you will pass less. If you take a big dose and not much comes out in your urine during the next day you must have needed a particular amount of that whereas if most of it does pass out during the next day, you actually have enough and you did not need it. It seems logical enough. It made sense to me.

However, after following through on all the data behind it, it turns out it is simply not accurate. The rate at which we eliminate iodine is rather constant through the urine but it takes many, many months to readjust after we are exposed to a big change. If we get much more or much less, it does not show up during a day. The other problem is if we are exposed to plenty of it, much of it goes through our bile and our stool or through our sweat. We get rid of unusually high doses through other mechanisms.

Therefore, the test is not accurate and the doses commonly recommended greatly exceed the doses that are safe for anyone, much less those who have thyroid disease. A common recommendation now by those faddish about iodine is to encourage doses anywhere from 6,000 to about 50,000 micrograms per day. The World Health Organization, after tracking volumes of data on iodine fortification, has shown most people can safely take about 1,100 micrograms per day. So again, recommended doses are 6-50 times above the safe upper limit for iodine.

In addition, iodine is probably the most studied mineral ever. The Chinese first learned back in about 2,500 BC that if they gave burned seaweed they could help people with a goiter or a swollen neck from thyroid issues. It was actually one of the first chemicals isolated in elemental form, one of the first nutrients known to have a specific function in the body, and we have tracked it closely for the last century. We have volumes of data on how much we need, what it does, when there is too much, when there is too little and clear data about its toxicity. We know exactly what happens when you get too much. With thyroid disease, the need for it is much smaller.

Now the paradox is you can develop thyroid disease from too little iodine. However, you can also develop it from too much. Because the amount of iodine we are normally exposed to is rather small, the body has a powerful mechanism that pulls iodine preferentially inside the thyroid. This lets the thyroid get first dibs on it, so to speak.

Now because that mechanism concentrates iodine so much, if we ever get too much iodine in our bodies, the gland has to shut itself off or it would make too much hormone, and dangerously so. That could make our heart give out – there would be so much thyroid hormone circulating. Whenever we get too much, it is toxic for our thyroid just as much as too little, if not more so. Moreover, if you have thyroid disease, which can occur even with amounts that would be healthy for someone else, especially if your dose changes rather abruptly. So as little as 300-400 micrograms above low intake can trigger issues for someone with thyroid disease, even if it has not been diagnosed or if it has not come to the surface just yet. So you do need iodine, but in tiny amounts.

Now another big thing to consider when you are on thyroid treatment is whether you are already taking iodine. Thyroid medicines inherently do contain a significant amount of iodine –typically about 0.2% in desiccated thyroid. Therefore, if you are taking a 1-grain dose of Naturethroid, for example, you are already getting 130 micrograms of iodine right there. That is about as much as you would need for the day if you have thyroid disease. Your diet naturally will contain a few hundred micrograms, even if you are not doing anything special – good or bad – so that and what you get in your thyroid is excellent – plenty. Aside from that, the principal goal is to avoid iodine. Better multivitamins do not include iodine. They actually make iodine-free versions for those who have thyroid disease. My personal favorite is Basic Nutrients V by Thorne, which is specifically made without iodine and iron, and is a good fit and a well-absorbed multivitamin as well. So overall, do avoid it.

Some products containing it are said to help the thyroid, especially specific iodine supplements such as Iodoral, potassium iodide, or Lugol's Iodine. I am torn by other thyroid support products because some of these products actually have otherwise good ingredients and they can be of some benefit, but you do have to watch their iodine content. Some have small enough amounts it can be negligible. Some of the better ones may have as little as 100 or so micrograms and if you are conscious of your intake from other sources this may not be a problem for you but there are products with an excess of 400 micrograms and this is amount is just not safe to add. It is just too much, despite whatever else you are doing if you have thyroid disease. So yeah, watch out for thyroid support products with more than 300-400 micrograms of iodine, and then definitely do iodine-free for multivitamins.

If you have thyroid disease, you are also better off using non-iodized salt and that is actually easy. Simply using sea salt, except for those few products already iodized, takes care of this. The benefit of sea salt is that it does have a significant amount of magnesium, which regular table salt does not. There are so many ways we can lack magnesium and benefit from it that it is worth adding any extra sources. So just do iodine-free sea salt daily for home use. Now we get most of our salt from processed foods and processed foods – they have tons of salt but it is generally non-iodized salt so for iodine – not as big a factor but aside from that – for a thousand other reasons – you do not want processed foods and plenty of salt anyway. So be on a low salt diet in general, and then use sea salt for what you do at home. It is better because of the magnesium content.

Now another important question that comes up often with a thyroid specific diet is of goitrogens. Goitrogens are specific things in plants, which change the chemistry of the thyroid gland and encourage the growth of a goiter.

If you have had a goiter or an enlargement of your gland this is more a factor for you. If you have not, it is less a factor. Now the paradox is that the goitrogens are found in plants that are generally healthy things for other reasons. The big category here are the cruciferous vegetables – broccoli, cauliflower, brussels sprouts, kale – these are plants rich in good chemicals. They can lower the risk of cancers and lower the risk of many other health problems, so it is better not to avoid them unnecessarily. The goitrogens are also fragile when exposed to heat especially when you are cooking your plants – cooking your veggies – typically not a big factor for you either. Not much to worry about.

One thing I do encourage monitoring and being aware of is your soy food intake. The goitrogens in general are from the cruciferous vegetables – their principal effect is to inhibit iodine absorption. If you are someone lacking iodine and consuming high numbers of uncooked cruciferous vegetables, you actually can create a hypothyroid state. Now the goitrogens in soy are somewhat different. These are isoflavones and they alter the activity within the gland rather than the absorption of iodine into the gland. Even if you have adequate iodine, soy can still inhibit your thyroid activity and it can create some inflammatory changes.

So if you are dialed in with does and your symptoms, your health and your weight, you know a dash of soy sauce here and there – some soy foods in your diet, especially the naturally fermented ones such as miso or tempeh, are not bad to have in your diet. However, if you are having a difficult time managing your weight, getting your dose right, then certainly you want to look for the more modern, processed versions of soy. These include soy protein isolates and all the versions of it found in foods are texturized vegetable proteins – good to be aware of and good to minimize.

However, other goitrogens – other plant foods – if they are lightly cooked they are fine to have in your diet and they are healthful foods for other reasons. Unless you are taking in several pounds of raw broccoli per day, it does not become a big factor. Generally, you are better off having the foods for their overall health impact than you are avoiding them for concern about possible thyroid effects. Again, the exception there is whether there is a goiter or enlargement or a difficult time getting dosing right.

A little more data on food allergies. For whom could this be an issue? With thyroid disease in general, screening at least once for food intolerances or food allergies is an intelligent step. We are talking about both intolerances and allergies. Allergies are IgE reactions. They are generally reactions that come on quickly and hit you hard and fast, and the relevance is they are not subtle. If you have them, you are probably already aware of it because you know if you eat a peanut, you cannot breathe for a while. It is a clear cause and effect, with dramatic symptoms coming on quickly. Now the intolerances – they are more gradual and more delayed.

Who do we think would have them? Well, people who are more prone to allergies in general. Some who have tendencies towards asthma, eczema, or known airborne allergens will have a higher rate of intolerances of all types. So they should be screened as well. However, for anyone with thyroid disease, it is intelligent to be screened at some point. If there are none showing up and your health is staying stable – nothing to worry about – no need to revisit. However, if they are present and they are numerous, it is intelligent to watch them annually just to see if there are changing, improving, and reducing. Ideally, they should.

There is a big overlap between how your intestinal tract functions and how your immune system functions. If the lining of the intestinal tract is irritated from chronic allergies or the wrong kind of bacteria, it is going to alter your body's entire immune system. It will make you more likely to be in a state of attack in your thyroid and make you more likely to develop more and more reactions and intolerances. So the better you avoid the reactive foods and being aware of them and the more your intestinal tract stays healthy, the milder all of these reactions become.

Chapter Summary

So many with thyroid disease have been confused about what to eat and what to not eat. The problem with this is that if you work hard to make changes that are not important, you will have less of an ability to make the changes that are important. Data has not shown gluten to effect the process of Hashimoto's Thyroiditis for those who do not have celiac disease. Some who have Hashimoto's do have gluten intolerances and they may have better digestive function without gluten. Yet even with gluten intolerance, gluten does not effect their thyroid function. The goitregens in soy and millet can have negative effects with Hashimoto's. Those found in cruciferous vegetables are more helpful than harmful. Weight loss can be prevented by the wrong balance of intestinal bacteria.

Action Steps

13. Consider IgG4 food intolerance testing

14. Minimize your intake of soy foods

15. Consume un-pasteurized Kimchee, sauerkraut, yogurt, kefir or use probiotics regularly.

Chapter 6

Hashis' Happens, Here's Why

Chapter At a Glance

- Toxins are the main cause of thyroid disease

- Toxins can also be the source of persistent symptoms and other health risks

- Total toxic burden

- Toxic fat

- General vs specific detox

- Testing for toxins

Detox your body. Toxins building up inside the thyroid cause thyroid disease. Consequently, detoxification is an essential step towards healing thyroid disease. If someone has persistent symptoms even after the dose is right, a big reason is the presence of the toxins that caused the disease first. They are often still in the body and causing many symptoms besides the thyroid disease.

So what is the role between toxins and thyroid disease? Well it is this. The thyroid gland has a sensitive mechanism that concentrates iodine. The body needs iodine for the thyroid to work but the amounts that we ingest are actually small. Most nutrients just diffuse throughout the body; the amounts in our bloodstream are enough for our needs. However, some nutrients are not in the blood in high enough amounts to suit our needs. The amounts in circulation are not always enough for certain tissues that need much more nutrient. Therefore, there are times when nutrients are concentrated and this is the case with the thyroid and iodine.

Therefore, what happens is that the thyroid has a mechanism that allows it to build more iodine inside itself than there is outside the rest of the body. It concentrates it strongly against a gradient. The iodine inside the thyroid may be present at a concentration fifty or one hundred times above what is in the rest of the body. It is good, because is needed. However, the problem is that many, toxins have a chemical similarity to iodine that is great enough to where they also get concentrated inside the thyroid. The same thing actually occurs to some extent in the brain. The brain is not concentrating iodine but it has a chemical property called the blood-brain barrier. What happens with the blood-brain barrier is that some things that enter the brain cannot always leave easily. Those chemicals diffuse into it but rather than flowing out, they are trapped inside and they tend not to leave so you end with concentrations in the brain much higher than they are in the rest of the body. The thyroid and the brain are both tissues that have numbers of toxins much higher than the rest of the body can carry. This is also why many with thyroid diseases have symptoms related to alteration in brain function, anxiety, depression, and short-term memory losses.

Over time, the presence of these toxins inside the thyroid starts to create an immune response. The body starts getting the immune cells activated, attacking these tissues carrying the toxins. The immune cells are secreting chemicals and antioxidants that would ideally help the breakdown and the removal of the toxins. In doing so, all the inflammation causes the cells to start getting reactive against the proteins present inside the thyroid gland. Often this dramatically worsens when the immune system is more active such as during an infection. Over time, we are sensitized to the gland. Therefore, that is how the disease starts but that is also what prolongs it. So the more wastes in the gland – even after the disease has already started – the greater the immune response will be. It has been shown clearly that even independent of your thyroid levels being right – as far as your dose being where it should be – and other factors being correct, the presence of high amounts of immune antibodies still can cause symptoms. The immune system is an important variable and one big factor that controls it is how many toxins are inside the gland.

To some extent, these issues come up for other autoimmune diseases – this presence of environmental toxins. We are exposed to more chemicals now than at any other point during human history. Some estimates have said more than three million new chemicals have been released in the environment since roughly the turn of the century. Moreover, the data is minimal as far as looking at the safety of them, how they work on the body, and how they are combined. At most a few percent have had thorough safety testing. We start our exposure before we are even born. In our mother's womb, many wastes cross the placenta, enter our bodies, and they can stay with us throughout our life span. Throughout our life, we are building up more and more toxins. More things are entering us.

In addition, a paradox that occurs is that the more we are exposed to, the more quickly things build up inside our bodies. What happens is the same small number of chemical pathways eliminates the many different toxins. Once we get a particular amount of toxic burden in our bodies, that finite number of chemical pathways is well blocked and we cannot eliminate much of anything.

So think about it like a clogged drain in a bathtub. You could have your bathtub overflow if the water was just totally on all the way and pouring out hard or you could have it overflow with just a drip over time – and that is kind of what can happen to our bodies. Once that drain becomes clogged – once we become less effective at detoxifying – then the small numbers of toxins we are exposed to everyday builds up with compounding interest. Eventually it hits a point where it is affecting us strongly and the sources of this are many.

We walk up and down the soap aisle. When we to the grocery store, things smell strong there because we are breathing a high number of solvents and fragrances. In our homes, we have carpeting. We have paints. We have fabrics and furniture and all these things are off-gassing formaldehyde and plastic residues. Our food is often carried in plastic and stored in plastic. We get exposure from this, these things go throughout our body, and they just continue building up in important parts of us. Some studies on some individual chemicals have been shown them to be harmful only when they are in amounts above our typical exposure levels.

However, there has been a newly emerging science showing that toxins act collectively much differently than they would act in isolation. This makes sense. If you put together blue and yellow, you get a new color. You get green. Chemicals do something similar to that too. When we have many different things, although they are in small amounts they do not act the way that any one of them would individually. The data we have on that is preliminary but well accepted. Recently the National Research Council (NRC) said that all the guidelines we have about toxins underestimate how they work together. The EPA and the FDA still only test the safety of chemicals individually. The NRC is saying that this is not meaningful because we have things that act collectively. We are exposed to not just isolated different things. It is many altogether and they build up.

These things affect us in many ways – not the least of which is they may be factors in the whole global obesity crisis. Here is the tie between toxins and obesity. Our bodies are known to bioaccumulate wastes in the tissues that have the least activity. They sweep toxins under the rug. We put things out of the way where we do not have to deal with them. One of the least critical tissues in our body we can do without is our fat tissue. If we have something dangerous that we cannot eliminate we will often bioaccumulate it in our fat. Later, when the body starts to break down fat, dangerous toxins are released. Fat breakdown is often slowed because our bodies cannot deal with the toxins. Therefore, the body will intentionally not break down fat stores when there is a high number of toxins in the fat. Of course, this is a big issue for those who have thyroid disease – the body weight issues and the weight gain. The toxins affect this directly by slowing the thyroid and making the body create antibodies against it. They also it affects our weight indirectly by slowing the breakdown of adipose tissue. So now, these things hit us in several ways.

We cannot escape exposure to toxins. We cannot avoid them completely. It has been shown that you can drill down a mile deep in the Antarctic and you can find DDT samples. So the stuff is everywhere to some extent. However, you can make a huge difference at lowering your total toxic burden and there are two steps to that. There is what comes in and what goes out. Thank about this again like an overflowing bathtub. We want it to not overflow and ruin the carpet. First, up we want to turn off what is coming in and the next step is we want to help what is going out go out faster.

The primary ways that we get things in are primarily through our diet, through what we are breathing and what absorbs across our skin. The principal way that things go out is through our body's elimination organs. How well we eliminate is based how effective our liver, our kidneys, our colon are working – also our skin and our respiratory tract. So the better we can eliminate and the less waste we can be exposed to, the lower our total toxic burden is. Some toxins do take more dedicated, specific measures to eliminate. They cannot come out as spontaneously or as easily – and we will talk about that as well. One difficulty is that if the body weight is fluctuating, that tends to take toxins out of the fat into circulation. If the body has poor ability to deal with them, then they tend to go right back in to deeper storage. At that point, it becomes more concentrated in the thyroid and in the brain.

So detox it – there are levels to it and ideally, it is pursued in a general way and a specific way. And by a "general way," that is there is a program I will outline – it is a good way once a year, especially in the spring – to help lower your total burden. The specific way is – those who have thyroid disease especially – it is wise to undergo particular testing to see what your burden is. This is done in several ways. There are direct tests and indirect tests. The direct ones just measure for actual toxins. This can be done through blood, urine, stool, and hair. Each of these methods has their strengths and weaknesses.

The blood tests are the most common in conventional medicine. They are accurate measurements of recent exposure, as in the last few days. Some troublesome type of toxins we are exposed to do not spend much time floating around in our blood. If they did, we would have a better chance at eliminating them. However, what happens is, because of their chemistry, they rather quickly migrate into our organs. This can include our thyroid, our brain, and our fat tissue. They are not in the blood for long periods. It is rather common that when we do a test on people, a conventional doctor may also see their laboratory reports. The other doctor will be surprised and say, "Wow, we wouldn't have suspected you had lead in your body. Let us retest this. Let us see if this shows up." Then the doctor will do a blood test, a serum lead test. Unless the patient was exposed to lead in the last several days, it will not be present.

The common serum tests – they are actually good if you are trying to see where someone is exposed. For example, say someone is known to have lead in the body from a more accurate test we will discuss. The serum test can be done at the end of the workweek, to see if the exposure might be at their job. If lead were not high during that time then we would not think of that as the source of exposure. Too commonly, these blood tests are done as the be-all and end-all – if they are even tested for at all. People just have them measured and doctors will say, "Oh no, you are fine. There is nothing here." Again, they only show the last couple of days of exposure. Blood tests have also been used for measuring such exotic things as some solvents and pesticides. The difficulty with those is similar. These also migrate rather quickly into stores. The other difficulty is there are not many laboratories that do these tests. A laboratory did more in the past that has gone by the wayside because it just was not used often enough. Consequently, many of these specific tests for pesticides and solvents are no longer available.

Toxicology tests are also done with urine. This can be done with or without a challenge. A "challenge" means something is given that would push toxins out of your body. In testing, this helps gauge what is in your deeper stores like your thyroid and your brain. The rationale is that some things, particularly metals, do get in your deeper stores but are not in a compartment like your blood or your urine normally that can be measured. So by giving a detox dose – by pushing some wastes out – you can then go on to do a measurement and evaluate what is in those deeper stores that was not coming out spontaneously. This is called a challenge test.

With the protocol, the common format is a compound that eliminates waste is given, then afterward a six or twenty-four-hour urine collection is taken. The idea is that these are wastes would not be spontaneously in the urine. You do not pee them out anyway, which is why they are stuck in your body first. Because they are not spontaneously in your urine – you are not getting rid of them – they stay in your body and they build up. So by giving a known challenge dose, then by seeing how much comes out after that dose then the lab and the doctor can work out exactly how much would be in that person's stores. If you do these tests, almost everyone has a little show up and there is probably a particular amount that is not significant.

In a perfect world, we would all be squeaky clean but there is likely a threshold below which the presence of some of these toxins is not significant. There are debates about where that threshold is but the reports do give levels categorized as normal and abnormal. When it is high, we can accurately say that there are more of those toxins in the stores than typical and that these toxins can be problematic for that person. If significant numbers of toxins do show up, the same intravenous solution can be given again to pull out the remaining toxins. Based on how high the score is, the doctor will recommend a particular number of treatments to be given. Ideally, the same test that was done at the beginning will be repeated with the last treatment to be sure the levels came down to the desired range.

In the challenge process – the most common compounds used are DMPS and EDTA. There is also an oral detox agent called DMSA that is commonly used. Overall, the detox agents are safe and well tolerated. There are those who do have allergies or sensitivities to them and there are those who have poor kidney function or other reasons that they should not undergo detoxification testing. Overall – well tolerated and no big negatives through the process. That is likely the most accurate way to gauge what the lifelong burden of metals is.

Hair is also used as a testing material and hair is somewhat handy in that it is non-invasive. It is also handy in that there are many laboratories that can do this test without the requirement of the doctor's order. You can buy a kit online from a laboratory, and they can mail a collection kit to you. In your home or with your stylist you can take an adequate amount of hair. Not much is required, usually a few tablespoons. This sample can be sent into the laboratory and analyzed.

The analysis of toxins in the hair from reputable laboratories is accurate. The shortcoming about the hair tests is that some laboratories have read too much into the data. They will claim to know a bit about more about your overall health and then can be determined from the hair alone. In some cases, it has received a bad rap because labs have made all kinds of conclusions that you could not make just from the hair.

Now the hair does have some correlation between what is in your body, obviously enough, but it is not always a predictable correlation. Therefore, with nutrients there are some nutrients tested in the hair. Generally, the panels that check for toxins do also measure for nutrients at the same time because they are all minerals. For some minerals tested for – what is in your hair is the opposite of what is in your body. More in your hair means less in your body and vice versa. A couple of big ones here are calcium and magnesium. Generally, if people have elevated levels of calcium or magnesium on a hair sample they have too little in their body and in their stores. Other nutrients have actually a good correlation between what is in your hair and what is in your body. Two that correlate accurately are selenium and manganese. So in general, the more of these you have in your hair, the more you have in your body and vice versa. There are many other nutrients where there is not a strong correlation between what is in your hair and what is in your body. Therefore, your hair levels could be high, low, or normal and your tissue levels could be high, low, or normal. It is not a strong predictor of them.

Now with toxins the hair generally does reflect the overall toxic burden of the body but not always linearly. So what that means... I think about hair tests almost like just positive-negative tests. I do not think about them for telling me how much somebody has in their body. I think about them as telling me whether some have significant numbers of toxins. If the hair says you have a high amount, you have probably some. It may not be a group but there is probably some, or it could be plenty. I would say the same thing if the hair says you have a moderate elevation. You may have some in your body. The hair tests are accurate in the cases in which they show that there is no significant toxic burden. Generally, if the hair test says there are no toxins in your body then there are probably none and it is not necessary to undergo further, more detailed testing. However, when the hair test says there are toxins in the body, there probably are but you cannot always say exactly by how much. Therefore, in those cases tests that are more detailed are helpful.

Now a newer thing to come available has been stool testing and many of the same things that I said about urine do apply to stool. This is part of our eliminatory pathway and certain wastes do show up in it. We are learning more that there may be a larger amount of some waste that passes through the bile and the stool than passes through the urine. There may be a little better accuracy. In addition, these are done with and without some provocation or a challenge. The negative is obvious. You have to make a prolonged collection of stool – usually twenty-four hours or more – and aside from just the obvious "ick" factor is that the difficulty is we do not have bowel movements on a predictably regular enough basis. Because of this, it may not reflect how much we eliminate over a set period. The volume of our urine from one day to the next – if you actually check all of it – is not radically different. But our bowel movements – some may miss a day and some may have several in the course of one day but not always the same amount of waste that we pass out of our bodies on a given day from one to the next. Therefore, that is a difficulty with the stool samples. We cannot determine how to compare one day with another. In addition, because of the collection factors they are not as widely used.

A couple more things available with some advanced versions of blood tests. The standard blood tests done by most doctors and reference laboratories are called serum tests. They are measuring the wastes in the watery portion of the blood called the serum and that is the area with the least duration of circulation in your body. It tends to be there for maybe a few days at the most.

However, some laboratories do tests on a few months' average amount of toxins attached to the red blood cells. This helps because the red blood cells are surviving and they are in circulation for roughly a three-month period. By measuring what they contain, that gives a better sense of what a longer-term average would be. It makes it more clear what would been circulating through the body for that period. Generally, the wastes we are concerned about, what they do is they come out of the stores, and they circulate. The principal stores are thyroid, the brain, the fat. There is a little breakdown, especially if it is fat tissue, on a day-to-day basis. As that breaks down the waste out of the fat goes through the circulatory process and ends by going to the organs of elimination. Usually, these wastes cannot be effectively eliminated. From there, then they go directly back into stores or they may be sent into the intestinal tract after which a large percentage is reabsorbed. They may go around, and then go back in again. However, as they do that a particular amount of them will become attached to the red blood cells and because the red blood cells are in circulation for about three months that gives a better picture of what your exposure could be than the simple serum tests would.

Now a difficulty here is that some things have a greater affinity for binding up with the blood than others do – so that too, should be taken into account. Arsenic, for example, has a high affinity for binding to the red blood cells. If we see some arsenic in the blood, we know that much of it is there and this is reflective more of the body's whole burden. Mercury is kind of the opposite. Mercury does not bind as readily to the red blood cells so if we see equal amounts of mercury and arsenic that would actually reflect a much higher burden of mercury because less of it does attach to these cells.

In addition, there are also whole blood element tests, which check the serum – the short-term exposure – plus the longer-term exposure from the blood cells and these are advantageous as well. The red blood cell tests and the whole blood elements tests are good because they can be done in a single blood draw. They do not require a challenge process.

Solvents and pesticides can also be present in the body. They are not accurately measured. There are not good tests for them. Usually, what happens though when they are present is to impair detox pathways causing more metals to bioaccumulate. So the metals are not only the principal clog of the drain but they are also the easiest part of that process to measure so they are the best area of focus in determining what people have in their systems.

Chapter Summary

Identifying and removing environmental wastes can help you feel better mentally and physically. It can help prevent and even reverse thyroid disease when it is at early stages. For many, toxins can also inhibit the success of their weight loss efforts.

Action Steps

16. Consider challenge testing for toxic metals

17. Undergo general detox annually. This can be as simple as a 10 day cycle of limiting all food to a detox meal replacement twice daily with 1 'lean and green' meal consisting of 4-6 ounces of fish or lean poultry + unlimited green vegetables. Mediclear SGS by Thorne is my favorite detox meal replacement.

Chapter 7

Getting Your Thyroid Squeaky Clean

Chapter At a Glance

- Value of organic foods

- Avoiding unnecessary chemicals in the diet

- Avoiding PCB's

- Mercury

- Plastic by products: BPA and PVC

- Clean air

The most critical step for effective detox is reducing the day to day burden, keeping what is coming in at a low threshold, and one of the larger sources of wastes to which we are exposed, would, of course, be our diets. In the diet, we are exposed to things primarily as by-products used in foods to help prevent pest growth or pesticide. We do also have a great deal of waste with just food processing and food storage so we get preservatives as well. Then by-products from containers and carriers of plastic derivatives – they will build up in foods. Overall, organic is not perfect. There are shortcomings and there are ways things said to be organic may truly not be. It can certainly happen that it can be mislabeled. There could be improvements with the regulations and with how foods are identified as organic.

Nonetheless, if you do switch to organic foods you will greatly lower your burden. That is one simple step. Overall, it would be wonderful if all our foods were organic but some things are a bigger factor than others are and in general, the foods that have had more exposure to the ground or the air are things that tend to have higher levels of pesticides. Therefore, that would include plants right on the ground – especially berries are common this way – things outside for longer periods can be problematic.

The best way to start reducing your chemical burden is to lower the number of toxins coming into the body. The biggest source of them is your diet with the biggest source of toxins consisting of processed foods and pesticides. Processed foods are simple to identify. This is anything that you would not have eaten on a farm one-hundred years ago. So commonly, people will ask about some particular ingredient or chemical and whether it is that dangerous or safe. Several individual ingredients have had some studies. However, we lack data on how they affect us when we consume different ones together. Even so, some are not as harmful, but they still require effort by your body's liver and detox organs to eliminate them. This lowers your overall ability to detoxify other substances and can increase your total toxic burden.

The easiest step to start with is by eliminating any chemicals you can. So do just minimize your chemical burden completely. Any vague ingredient that would not have appeared on the farm a century ago – do not eat it. In addition, if there is an ingredient list a paragraph long – do not even bother reading it. Just put it back. An extremely good trend lately has been the whole clean-eating revolution. It is just common sense – good advice. Eat simple foods – things in a minimally processed state. This includes meat, fish, poultry, produce, grains – ideally intact, whole grains – beans, nuts and seeds, some dairy foods and eggs. Simply avoiding packaged and pre-made foods can lower your chemical burden substantially. One of the things you do not always hear is that the chemicals in foods also play tricks with our apatite. Food producers add artificial flavorings and ingredients knowing that they will make you want to eat and buy more than you need.

The next step in lowering your chemical burden from your diet is to avoid pesticides. The largest source by far is produce. Ironically, produce is also the richest source of plant chemicals that help our bodies with detoxification. If you are not getting half of your food volume from produce, doing so should be your first focus.

Something I want to warn you about quickly. If you read plenty of health advice, there is a dangerous process I call "the perfect being the enemy of the good. " That is where we can learn so many ideals or rules or such lofty goals that we can end by just feeling overwhelmed, then you know – eat Doritos – not worry about any of it because there is so much to take into account. Always make the best choices you can with whatever you have. When you do have the option then make the even better choices. However, if produce is available for a snack – even if it is not organic – that is going to be a better snack than a processed food would be. So keep that in context. Think about things more as a hierarchy than just good and bad. The better food is produce and better food yet is organic produce.

Worry more about getting more produce than choosing organic. If you are already doing well at getting produce, then start thinking about choosing organic to replace that produce with the highest number of pesticides. A current list of the highest sources of pesticides can be found on the Environmental Working Group's "Dirty Dozen" list: www.ewg.org.

The current list includes apples, bell peppers, carrots, celery, cherries, grapes, kale, lettuce, nectarines, peaches, pears, and strawberries. So those particular ones, you do want to go out of your way to find organic sources. The ones not on that list, they are not as big a factor.

Another factor is keeping your produce clean. You want to wash it thoroughly. There still will be some types of toxins and wastes even on the organic produce. There is no way to avoid that totally. So give it a thorough scrub. Wash your produce in a sink full of cold water with one cup of vinegar added. This can reduce the load of waste and chemicals and irritants and even some bacteria by high amounts. Something you can do also to reduce the number of pesticides on non-organic things is to soak them in a container with the vinegar for a period. So roughly a cup of vinegar to a large sink of water and let things soak for about ten or twenty minutes and after that time give them a little scrub. Other things you can just drop them in and just soak completely – things like grapes or cherries. They can just sit in that solution for up to an hour and that can greatly decrease the pesticide residue.

There are other foods inherently much lower in pesticides. With these, you would not need to worry about going out of your way to get organic. These are called the "clean dozen" and include asparagus, avocados, cabbage, eggplant, kiwis, mangoes, onions, papayas, pineapples, sweet corn, sweet peas, and watermelon. So these particular ones – do not bother spending the extra money on getting organic because they do not tend to have waste in them to begin with.

We are exposed to other toxins besides pesticides. One group of these is compounds called polychlorobiphenyls (PCBs). They are especially good to be aware of because they are toxic to the brain and nervous system. They are found in a big variety of foods. One of the biggest ones, unfortunately, is farm-raised salmon. We know that fish is a good source of omega-3 fats and it is important to have in the diet. PCBs are toxic and they have actually been shown to have strong effects upon how well children's brains develop. However, you do want wild salmon over the farm raised, primarily because of the PCB content. Thankfully, salmon is not a large source of mercury like other types of fish.

Now along the lines of fish, we want to think about mercury from other types as something to avoid. The easiest rule of thumb with that is the larger the fish are, the longer they have lived and the more time they have had to build up mercury in their flesh. Unfortunately mercury is part of just the whole ocean's biosphere so all ocean life carries some mercury. Once the mercury gets into living systems' tissues, it never leaves. It continues to build up. Imagine that a tiny fish has a low concentration of mercury in its tissue, say one part per billion. Slightly larger fish eat them and concentrate the mercury further, say to one part per million. Even larger fish eat them and may concentrate it to one part per hundred thousand.

So the higher and higher you go up the food chain, the more mercury things contain.

Specifically the biggest problem with fish and mercury is tuna, and the reason is that many people eat it as a food frequently. There certainly are types of fish that have more mercury than tuna but most of them are ones people do not eat that frequently. That is going to be things like swordfish or thresher shark. Tuna would be a good source of protein and omega-3 fats but the mercury does bioaccumulate. Most adults can safely consume between four and six ounces of it daily.

Besides being aware of the chemicals in your food, also think about the containers into which you are putting your food. We are exposed to so much plastic and plastic does give off many compounds, including phthalates and bisphenol-A (BPA) Thankfully recent regulation will eventually limit our BPA exposure. However, some still exists in the environment to which we are exposed. Therefore, it is still there. One of the worst ways you can process foods with plastic is to microwave them. When you heat things in plastic, the amount of all those wastes just penetrates the food. This makes the toxins that much more absorbable and that much more able to build up in the body. Then of course, be aware of plastic wraps. If you put plastic wraps over food and microwave them, it will cause even more of a buildup in the system.

The most toxic plastic is polyvinylchloride (PVC). You can identify this by recycling codes #5 and #6.

Another toxin to be aware of is Styrofoam. Coffee in Styrofoam cups gives off amounts of xanthenes and other toxins such as polycarbonate. These have been shown to raise rates of both obesity and cancer. Some less toxic ones based upon the recycling labels numbers one through four. Those generally have less of an impact.

Remember with plastics, lower recycling numbers are safer.

Are you still with me? Are you starting to think the world is dangerous and out to get you? I promise it is not but when you are learning to spot invisible dangers it can first feel that way!

Another big source of toxic exposure from the diet will be from fats – from animal fats especially. I mentioned before how we are exposed to wastes and they build up in our fat tissues. It is the same with the animals we eat. So when we are consuming dairy, beef, poultry, pork or other animal foods, the higher the fat content, the greater the amount of pesticide residue.

Therefore, for animal foods that contain fat, they are higher priority foods to find in organic forms. The leaner they are the less a factor this is but the amount of fat present makes the amount of pesticide load higher. Butter, for example, is one of the foods that you want to prioritize for an organic version. Some non-fat versions of milk or white meat poultry – that is less a priority. However, things that contain animal fats are a high priority for getting organic.

Another source of day-to-day exposure for wastes is going to be the air we breathe. An easy step for this is to keep a good HEPA filter in your bedroom – where you spend most of your time. That will take the waste down by a substantial amount. Minimizing fabric in the home is also helpful. If you do have a home that has been recently built or painted, or you have new furniture or carpets, the often noticeable odor is not only unpleasant, but also dangerous. These are all VOCs or volatile organic compounds. Thankfully, there are more options with paints lower in this or free of VOCs but it is still an issue for many new things, especially carpets.

Carpets also give off formaldehyde in high amounts. An option for that is one-time use of a high-powered ozone generator. These can be purchased or rented. You run them in the house or the room for between twenty-four and forty-eight hours while you are away. They make amounts of ozone that effectively break down the chemicals that would be dangerous to be exposed to. The idea is you would run this device as you were out and let it break down the chemicals, and then you could come back after typically a day or so of it being off. They usually have timers that can have them run for twenty-four hours and you want to be away while it was running and long enough for the whole reactions to stop. That makes a considerable difference in reducing the noticeable odor but also reducing the number of circulating chemicals in the air and in the environment.

Chapter Summary

We are swimming in an ocean of man-made chemicals everyday. The vast majority have never undergone safety testing in isolation. None have undergone adequate safety testing for the combinations in which we are routinely exposed. Small everyday choices can serve to lower our toxic exposure dramatically.

Action Steps

18. Change to organic for high priority foods

19. Eat simple foods. If a food was not present prior to the 1930's, don't eat it.

20. Reduce your chemical burden at home with green cleaning products and air filters.

Chapter 8

Best and Worst Pills for Your Thyroid

Chapter At a Glance

- Don't be a 'new pill' junkie

- Essential supplements for anyone

- Do we get the RDA?

- Tablets vs capsules

- Which excipients and binders to avoid

- Role of assimilation

- Folic acid conversion

- Essential fats

- Calcium the double edged sword

- Vitamin D

Supplements for people who have thyroid disease. Which should you take, which should you not take, and why does it matter? We will clear all of that up.

With taking pills, people come in two types. Some take whatever they are told is new and exciting. They have a long list of pills they take. Often they are most familiar with those that have appeared most recently. Online doctors, websites, or newsletters are usually marketing these. They might not be taking things that have been around for long periods or they might not be thinking about them because they are not as exciting.

The other big group is those who do not take pills, because they do not like to or they are not regular about it. A few people share a little of each. They like to buy pills but they do not take them well. Maybe you have your own little health-food store started at home in your closet or in your pantry. I have got a bit of overflow in myself, to be honest.

Here is the thing. Only a particular number of pills will be taken regularly on a day-to-day basis. The odds of someone taking large numbers of pills consistently are extremely small.

It is important to figure out what is critical and most helpful, and then focus on that. If you do dilute your pill list with a whole lot of things that may not be as critical for your needs then you will not take the important ones. There are some things that you do strongly want to avoid as well, and we will go into that in good detail.

A quick overview. I break supplements into those that anyone who has thyroid disease should be taking and those that might help some people. The last group is those that have a few possible benefits but perhaps not much data behind them. I do not encourage taking these possibly helpful items, because you might not take many other items you should be taking.

The real core things that most of us do need come down to multivitamin, fish oil, calcium, magnesium and vitamin D, and we will go through all those in detail and talk about other things that may be useful as well.

You hear this so many times that a well-balanced diet should supply all the vitamins and minerals for adult health. It has to be true because you have heard it so much. However, the sad fact is it is far from true. I taught nutrition for several years in a medical school just after I graduated. I was working hard and getting the practice going and taking secondary jobs like that to help make ends meet. That was one, and I enjoyed it.

One exercise in these nutritional classes that I found so enlightening to the young doctors was to devise a diet that would meet the recommended dietary allowance of their nutrients.

People think RDA means daily allowance. Actually, it does not as it means dietary allowance. The distinction is that it is meant to be a week's average. It is understood that some days you will get less of something but the expectation is you will make up for that elsewhere throughout the week. There is just this strong belief that somehow or other just eating random foods that we have in our modern world you are going to cover all the bases for your nutrients.

In the exercise, what I had them do is to first log their diets for a week, then we would run mathematics, on vitamins and minerals. We would see how much of which they got. There is software for this nowadays that makes this easy, but back then there was not. We had the giant books that listed thousands and thousands of foods and gave exhaustive tables for each in how much nutrient any food had. We would go through all this, and then add them. Lo and behold their diets were low in many, many key nutrients - calcium, magnesium, vitamin C were commonly lacking. Some B vitamins would be as well. Other key minerals were commonly lacking.

The next step was to devise a diet that will meet all the needed nutrients from the recommended dietary allowance, during a week to meet this average. The expectation was that if you plan the scheme knowing what your low spots were you could do it. Now, the one rule I set on them was they had to devise a diet that had a reasonable caloric load. You cannot just do ten-thousand calories per day to get adequate amounts of a particular nutrient. It has to be a realistic diet.

With that scheming, planning, and looking at books and charts, they realized it was impossible, that you cannot hit all the needed nutrients even on a devised diet. Once someone goes through that exercise and sees that firsthand they start taking multivitamins. There is just no two ways about that.

Now, multivitamins do vary from type to type. Here are some key factors to look for. Some nutrients do not absorb that well when they are taken with other nutrients. Probably the biggest one that is complicated to absorb well is iron.

So, if iron is taken with other things, other minerals will not absorb well. The iron will not absorb at all well and the antioxidants are going to be broken down. What happens to an iron gate if you leave it out somewhere coastal or somewhere that is humid? It is going to rust, right? Rusting is free radical damage, which is the same as happens on a molecular basis to iron when mixed with other things inside a pill. The antioxidants are used up, it rusts, and it oxidizes.

The first step for a multivitamin is you do want one that is iron free. Another big step and probably the most compelling reason to take a multivitamin, especially for those who have thyroid disease - is you want to get those important trace minerals, things like the selenium, the manganese, the zinc, the chromium, the copper. They are so critical and they are commonly lacking in the diet.

Now, to get them in your system you are going to need to break them down properly and absorb them well. One big barrier for absorption is tablets. You do not want tablets. People always say, "Should I take this pill?" I do not even open the bottle. I just shake the bottle. If you hear the hard rattling of tablets inside the bottle, throw the pill away because with multivitamins especially they will not break down effectively to give you those trace minerals. Therefore, you want capsules.

Now, here is another factor to consider. With capsules, there is a variety of excipients and binders and dispersers. These are all things that allow the powder to flow through the machines smoothly and effectively. That allows the machines to make literally three times the number of capsules they can make if there was not soap and slippery things mixed in the powder. It is a big advantage for manufacturers to add things to the powder so it can go into the capsules quicker and through the machines quicker. They can make more per day with the same amount of factory space and factory time.

The problem is that many of these ingredients are just not good for us. We see this so often – things that are handy to add to foods might not be healthful for us – such as food colorings, trans fatty acids, processed sugars, extra salt, preservatives, among others. Many things are convenient for manufacturers but do not work well in the human body. One of the biggest here is magnesium stearate, a kind of soap that makes the molecules of whatever nutrient more slippery and less capable of keeping themselves together. Maybe it is good for the machine but they will slip straight through your intestine track into the toilet. They will not do you any good. You want to avoid magnesium stearate. Look at the list of inactive ingredients, and if the product does not list the inactive ingredients then do not even bother with it. Magnesium stearate can also be present when products list ascorbyl palmitate or stearic acid.

Now, a couple of pitfalls. Some low-quality companies do not even list what additives or excipients they use. Therefore, if they do not even list the secondary or inactive ingredients then you might as well put it back as there is going to be a load of junk in there.

I did a video experiment in which we added baking soda to vinegar. If you have ever seen a volcano at a science fair then it creates an exothermic reaction. It foams, making an exciting, fizzy mess. However, if you add only 1% magnesium stearate to the baking soda and drop it in the vinegar, nothing happens. It sits there like a clump of just inert powder, and then it drops to the bottom if you try to stir it in. Amazing, as little as 1% completely neutralizes a dramatic chemical reaction. You can just imagine what the same amount or more does to the delicate absorption of microscopic vitamins and minerals inside your intestinal tract. It makes them worthless. If you are going to take pills, you want to absorb them.

There is a saying, "You are what you eat." However, you are what you assimilate. You can visualize the intestinal tract as a big tube. Imagine you have a six-inch wide tube from your mouth to your rectum. If you dropped a pill in that tube, it could fall through and right out the other end, and never interface with your body meaningfully. The gut is actually like that. It happens to be much longer, has a few more twists and turns, is much smaller, however, it is not dissimilar to that tube. What has to happen is the nutrients have to cross the lining. They have to get into the bloodstream and magnesium stearate is one of the big issues of making nutrients not absorb properly, so you do want to avoid that.

Another big factor for multivitamins with people that have thyroid disease is iodine. Now, iodine is commonly added to many multivitamins. Some companies do make multivitamins without iodine and iron. It is worth looking for. The negative about iodine is that you want to keep your intake low to minimize your thyroid antibodies. Dietary sources are almost negligible. You do want to avoid iodized salt and I would encourage avoiding kelp and other seaweeds high in iodine, like Dulse and Wakame. The amount in Nori is small enough to be negligible if it is eaten a few times a week. That is the green stuff wrapped around sushi. I love sushi; it is good stuff and Nori is tasty. Thankfully, its iodine load is negligible.

When you are taking thyroid medications - synthorid, levoxil, cytomel, desiccated thyroid, you are getting iodine. The medications and the active hormones inside the medications are iodine based. T4 means four iodine atoms for every T, every tyrosine. You are getting iodine already in your thyroid replacement. Therefore, if you want to keep your iodine load low to minimize your antibody score, you have to watch out for your other sources, so it is certainly not a good idea to take multivitamins that have iodine.

A couple more things to look at – Folic acid, for example. An enzyme activates folic acid. B vitamins often are not useful until your body converts them into secondary chemicals, and this primarily occurs inside the liver. Folic acid is converted to a substance called five methyltetrahydrofolate – try saying that three times fast. Not me, because it is boring. We call it MTHF for short and that is what folic acid is converted into by your body.

Now, many people do not do a good job converting folic acid, and then they can consume it from food or supplemental sources and still be lacking the active effect of folic acid, however much folic acid they ingest, because they are not converting it. Guess what – those that do not convert well are part of a group common for people who have thyroid disease. The better multivitamins have folic acid as five methyltetrahydrofolates, or MTHF, and that is important.

Another thing is that biotin; you do want a good dose of biotin. Biotin is important for your hair regrowth, and that is a factor for many that have thyroid disease. Your thyroid hormones, if they are not in the right amount they dictate how well your connective tissues grow. The first place that takes the hit there is going to be hair, skin, and nails, and we know we need biotin for those.

Here is a little insider's scoop on the supplement industry. They put many specific ingredients on there to make it look like you are getting quite a number of vitamins in general, then they skimp on a few others. Why would that be? Well, that is because of raw-material costs. With things such as thiamin, riboflavin, and some B vitamins, the raw-material cost is cheaper than dirt – cheaper than the bottle. They put many of those in there so it looks as though, "Wow, I'm getting 500% of the RDA, or often 5,000%. They must be putting plenty of good things in here." When you look at the biotin content, it might be only 10% or 30% of the RDA. What is wrong with that?

Biotin is important. Biotin is not toxic. The only reason that they skimp on biotin is that it is the most expensive raw material they use. In addition, they are cutting corners where they can so they are skimping on your biotin. So make sure you are getting at least three-hundred micrograms of biotin in the multi, otherwise you would need it separately and suddenly your multi would not become cost-effective. You would be justified in getting a better-quality one.

Trace minerals, you want the trace minerals there as it is one of the main reasons you are taking a multivitamin to begin with. I would look for the inclusion of selenium, manganese, and vanadium. A few newer ones such as vanadium, molybdenum, and chromium are important for those who have thyroid disease. Some include it, some do not, but you want to make sure they are in there.

The second most important thing to be taking is fish oil. If you are eating fish three times a week, you are probably getting adequate amounts of omega-3 fats in your diet, and that is wonderful. However, you want to push your body to an anti-inflammatory state. So do eat the fish. However, some benefits of fish protein may not translate in the fish oil, therefore, you do want to eat fish, and you want to take fish oil.

You want to get those do not have contaminants, you want to get those with high amounts of EPA and DHA, and you want to get those with a little vitamin E to prevent the oils being oxidized or getting free radical damage.

You can get these in capsules or in oil. In general, capsules tend to be a bit more stable. Oils tend to be a bit more cost-effective. Most people prefer capsules because of convenience in taking but both can work fine. One trick is that if you are getting oil you can add that into a smoothie. The better-quality fish oil is minimally enough of a fish taste to where you can get a small amount in a smoothie and do fine with it, so that is an option. Gel caps can be taken easily, and they can be mixed into a smoothie. The better-quality ones nowadays, they will use tilapia itself or fish protein for forming the capsule and that dissolves readily inside a blender. So you can drop those in and add in some protein powder and some frozen fruit. You will barely even know it is there and it will go down well and absorb effectively.

With fish oil, there is a considerable difference from one to the next in how much omega-3 fat you get per serving, and especially how much EPA you get per serving. So look around. The better-quality ones will give you at least 70% or so of omega-3 fats, which means most products are thousand-milligram gel caps. For each one-thousand milligrams of fish oil, they will say how much actual EPA and DHA that you receive from that. You add those two and you can calculate the percentage of omega-3 fats. For example, if it says a thousand-milligram gel caps giving you two-hundred and fifty milligrams of EPA and two-hundred and fifty milligrams of DHA, or five-hundred milligrams of omega-3 fats, you can just knock off that zero and that is 50% EPA – a little on the low side, as ideally, you should be getting 70% or more essential fats out of the fish oil.

The relevance of that is twofold. One is that you can take fewer pills and still be on a good dose, and that is super handy. The other relevance is that there is a whole lot less random fish junk that you may not need because it has been molecularly distilled and concentrated. You do want pharmaceutical grade – that is a term to look for – and you want to ensure the company has some independent testing for toxins. That is something that is important to have. Just know that testing is not always done that well, so the better concentration you have of EFAs - essential fatty acids - the less room there is for contaminants. It should not be oxidized, which you can tell by the taste as oxidized oils taste rancid or bitter and fishy. The good-quality ones have minimal flavor to them at all so that is a good thing.

Another thing that anyone should take daily, especially those with thyroid disease, is going to be calcium. Calcium, this is a huge source of controversy and confusion, unbelievably. If you followed the news, over the last year there have been many stories about vitamins causing death and it is true. The media have handled this in a somewhat irresponsible way, but that is how they put the stories out. In the big scheme of things, statistically, specific things do raise the risk of death. In the big scheme of things, the number of people dying of properly used medications now is barely exceeded only by cancer and heart disease. However, to think that vitamins are our nemesis is quite misleading. We also have about 30,000 emergency room visits monthly from simple things like aspirin and Tylenol and acetaminophen. It just happens that synthetic medications have a much higher toxicity profile than natural compounds or vitamins do.

Even so, there is plenty of poor-quality calcium available in the market and what happens is that calcium can go a couple of different directions in the body. Calcium can calcify or it can mineralize. By calcify I mean that it is going to form calcified junk. That can contribute to gall stones, kidney stones, calcified plaque in the arteries, or calcifications in the joints. Specific types of calcium in the blood can worsen inflammation and the build-up of junk – mostly insoluble calcium, or calcium that does not readily absorb in water. That type of calcium is again to the benefit of the manufacturer as it has a lower material cost and a greater concentration. Therefore, for less money and fewer pills, they can give you more milligrams of calcium when they use an insoluble type of calcium. However, the difficulty is that it is going to calcify, which is why you see people who take higher amounts of calcium have more cardiovascular deaths.

Therefore, you need soluble calcium, which has the advantage of not requiring high amounts of stomach pH to absorb. The insoluble forms of calcium do not work well if your digestion is poor, or if you are taking acid blockers. The main soluble types are calcium citrate and better yet calcium citrate maleate. Other factors are that other types of calcium also have a great tendency towards having lead contamination. We see this with oyster shell calcium, with calcium carbonate, which is what Tums is, and with bone based calcium as well as C-based calcium. Some products, such as those derived from bone, are marketed as having superior absorption. They actually can absorb well but the bad thing is they do have lead in them.

A big example of this is microcrystalline hydroxy apatite (MCHA), also called microcrystalline hydroxy apatite complex (MCHC). MCHA also has a tendency toward being contaminated with lead, so there are some negative factors to that. Then we have sea-derived calcium, and you might remember the big buzz about coral calcium many years back. Coral calcium was taken off the market because of crazy high claims, but also because of issues of purity.

The next version is what is called plant derived or algae derived calcium, which is being introduced on the market by many big companies. Guess what – it is repackaged and relabeled coral calcium – and popular with manufacturers because it is a cheap raw material and they can get a good profit margin with it.

This theme often comes up as supplement companies want to take something cheap and sell it for a high price. They want cost-effective raw materials such as sea-derived and the insoluble types of calcium. However, they are good to avoid. With calcium, it is important to get the right types.

Magnesium is an important one for anyone, too. Although there are not as many complications with magnesium, you do still want the citrate and the citrate maleate types for the best purity. One thing to be aware of with magnesium is that it does have laxative properties. Sometimes this is helpful, especially for those who have chronic constipation because of thyroid disease – magnesium is one of the most effective ways to reverse that, and it is safe.

Laxatives can work by stimulating the colon to move – that is called a stimulate laxative. Alternatively, they can work by carrying more water through the colon – that is called an osmotic laxative. The stimulant laxatives are usually plant-based laxatives, such as senna, cascara sagrada, or rhubarb. These are commonly taken as they cause you to have a rather strong bowel movement within several hours – and they work – but the problem is with regular use it requires more of a dose to achieve the same effect, so they are habit forming for the body. If you stop them you can get bad constipation, and over long periods they actually stain the colon and they start creating malabsorption tendencies, so they are good to avoid.

Magnesium, however, is an osmotic laxative and it is safe to use daily. You can take as much a dose as you need and your bowels will work fine and you will not get habit-forming tendencies from it. For most folks, it goes the exact opposite. They take it daily and if they stay regular, over time they end by needing less and less, a good sign.

For some people magnesium can be a bit of an irritant for the intestinal tract, aside from its laxative effects. It is better to take with food, and generally, it seems to work better if it is in a ratio of one-to-one or about one and a half parts calcium to magnesium, meaning you want a little more calcium than magnesium or roughly equal amounts.

The last thing I would encourage for everyone would be some version of vitamin D. Vitamin D is unique in that we know exactly how much you need in your blood. The downside is that how much dose of vitamin D it takes to achieve the targeted blood levels ends up being quite different from one person to the next. The other factor with vitamin D, it is a fat-soluble vitamin, so it does bioaccumulate or builds up in the body. There has been quite a bit of media about the benefits of it and I see many folks who actually take far too much. Many people take five-thousand or ten-thousand units, day in, day out, long term. Over time, this can be commonly excessive. However, the difficulty is some need that much to get to a decent range. Therefore, the intelligent thing with vitamin D does take some monitoring.

The preferred blood test is called the serum 25 hydroxy vitamin D. Ideally we see that score in the 40-65 nanogram per mil range. It could take none for some folks that have quite a bit of sun exposure, or it could take ten-thousand units a day to get someone loaded up if they are low in it.

Now, a few issues of sun exposure. The obvious one is the risk for skin cancer if it is excessive, so you want to be mindful of your complexion, your personal history, and your family history.

The other factor that makes it unreliable is we do not get exposed that much, that often. We are covered, we wear clothes, and we wear sunscreen. However, here is the big kicker. There are oils that allow our skin's pigment melanin to help synthesize, form, and assimilate vitamin D. In addition, these oils take many days to form. So daily bathing, a good idea – I am sure you do already, if not, an intelligent thing to think about. However, good, regular, daily bathing unfortunately makes your skin less able to absorb vitamin D. So if we were naked, dirty cavemen walking around - cavemen and cavewomen, mostly cavewomen probably in the audience - if we were like that and we were outside exposed to quite a bit of sun in more equatorial areas we would not be vitamin D deficient. However, the reality is most of us are not in equatorial areas. We are wearing clothes, we are bathing, we are probably even wearing some sunscreen and covering up, and that leaves us deficient.

In medicine, we have known forever that if you are low in vitamin D your bones will not grow healthy and there is a tendency towards osteoporosis for adults and rickets for kids. It does not take a ton of vitamin D to offset that problem. The presence of it helps proper absorption of calcium and proper mineralization of calcium. We have talked about how calcium can calcify or mineralize. That is a function of what type of calcium we consume and how much of it, but it is also a function of our vitamin D status. So if we are lacking vitamin D, whatever calcium we ingest is more apt to calcify and create junk and scar tissue and stones in the body and less apt to mineralize and create healthy, strong bone tissue. Therefore, we need adequate vitamin D for that, too, as the amounts can be variable.

Another issue with vitamin D is absorption. It is fat-soluble but it is not as readily absorbed as some nutrients. So generally, when you are taking it you do want it with food. Many things can go with and without food. With Vitamin D, you do want it with food and you want some kind of fat with that meal, some kind of healthy fat - nuts or seeds, avocados, some healthy oils, perhaps an egg. However, you want some fat with that meal to get the vitamin D in your system.

The amount you need for offsetting bone disease is quite small. Most can do okay with even four-hundred units per day not to have osteoporosis or rickets. However, we are learning with vitamin D, those in the higher range – way above what would cause bone issues – have much lower rates of all kinds of chronic diseases. This is shown to be relevant to cardiac disease, for many cancers, for dementia, for Parkinson's, for Alzheimer's, for kidney disease. So it turns out there is a sweet spot for vitamin D, a decent measure above the amount that offsets osteoporosis.

Now, papers have shown that there is also a high range and if you are above a particular range, there are higher rates of total mortality. We are not sure what the exact reasons or mechanisms, but we know that too much is also not good. You want to be in that sweet spot for vitamin D. This easy trick can help you achieve longevity. So have a measurement done for a baseline. If you are already there check it regularly, on an annual basis. If you are not there, it takes a little while for the blood levels to respond to a change in dosage, usually about six months. If someone is low in it, most adults can do well to start with five-thousand units a day, then have a reassessment done to confirm they are back at a healthy range. If they are, anywhere from two-thousand to three-thousand units is the common dosage to stay stable. These are common guidelines, but I see folks range from one-thousand to ten-thousand units per day with what helps and keeps them at a good range.

Now, with vitamin D, another factor with your multivitamin I would encourage is to make sure you are getting adequate amounts of vitamin K, too. That is important for calcium going the right way when vitamin D brings it in. Those things all work together. So be sure your multivitamin does give you the full RDA amount of K, too.

That much rounds out the main things that everyone should take. In this next section, we will go into more specific thyroid helpers that can do good things for those who have thyroid disease.

Chapter Summary

Supplements are needed to get optimal amounts of essential nutrients. Unfortunately, many people spend their time and efforts taking supplements that are not necessary or not effective. There are many aspects of manufacturing that can make supplements not absorb or work properly. People with thyroid disease do have distinct needs when it comes to supplementation.

Action Steps

21. Avoid tablets, use capsules. Liquid supplements sound like a good idea but end up having too many flavorings and preservatives to be effective.

22. Avoid ingredients like magnesium stearate that may impair nutrient absorption.

23. Consider testing your genes for folic acid conversion or take pre-converted folic acid also called 5-MTHF.

24. Avoid insoluble calcium, do take soluble calcium.

25. Test Vitamin D levels to be sure you're getting enough and not too much.

Chapter 9

Healing Your Adrenals

Chapter At a Glance

- Adrenals are the 'sister glands' of the thyroid

- Circadian regulation

- Many roles of the adrenals

- DHEA and pregnenolone

- Stress control

- Adrenal and thyroid interactions

- Cortisol and melatonin

- Adrenal testing

- Adrenal treatments

If someone has been doing all the right things – they are on a good diet, they have got their hormones in a good range, they are taking the appropriate supplements – and they are still not feeling right, well what do we think about it? One thing that comes up often would be the adrenal glands. There is a large overlap in function between the thyroid and the adrenal glands. Many jobs do both, and commonly when one gland – such as the thyroid – is not working correctly, the other gland – the adrenals – can often be altered somehow because of that. As a generalization, whenever one is taxed the other tends to be taxed as well. So they are good to consider and think about whether someone is still symptomatic – and we will talk about them in good detail to know what they do and what their role is and how to understand how they are working and most important, how to correct it and get you feeling better.

Just as we have learned that with the thyroid, for the adrenals, testing can be superficial or thorough. The adrenals make a large range of hormones. To add to the complications, some hormones they make vary at various times of day. The fluctuation from one person to the next can be substantial but also from people to themselves, just from one time of day to the next, can also have a considerable difference. Because of this, doctors have been hesitant to get too involved in looking at subtle changes. They have only focused on the big changes when the glands are completely overactive or when they are completely shut. So let us get an overview here of what they are and what they do.

The adrenal glands are two little lumps of tissue, usually triangular pyramid shape, and they sit on top of your kidneys. They are also called suprarenal glands which means "above kidney" and that is their location. However, their job is not the same as the kidneys. There can be tissue from the adrenal glands in other parts of the body as well. Erratic amounts of hormone are made because it is not properly regulated in that condition. Especially if someone has unexplained high blood pressure, intense anxiety, or palpitations, we have to think about there being adrenal tissue outside its proper home as a possible culprit.

The adrenal glands have three layers inside them. The outside layer makes a hormone called aldosterone and that regulates how much salt and water you carry in your body. That is a big part of how we keep our blood pressure in proper check and properly regulated. The middle layer makes primarily cortisol and forms a big part of regulating your blood sugar but it does a bit more. It also does affect inflammation. It does also have an effect on your thyroid hormones. Adequate amounts of cortisol are needed for thyroid hormones to be used by the cells. Too much cortisol, however, can block the inner portions of the cell from using thyroid hormones. Either too much or too little cortisol can disrupt the thyroid. The innermost portion, a little deeper than the area that makes cortisol, makes hormones such as testosterone and estrogen. It is job is to make reproductive type hormones. The testicles and the ovaries make these hormones primarily, but there are versions of them also made here by the adrenal glands. The innermost portion makes adrenaline, a hormone that is an instant instigator of the whole fight-or-flight response. Therefore, these various layers have different jobs.

Now something somewhat unusual happens when there is a stress on the gland or if it is not working right, what can happen is that one portion of the gland can swell dramatically and that can put pressure on other portions of the gland and that can actually create some localized pain or discomfort. So we think about that if someone has symptoms suspicious of there being adrenal problems and non-specific back pain but no real history of back trauma or accidents or musculoskeletal issues or arthritis. There could be simple impingement from the adrenals causing it.

The principal hormones made are pregnenolone, cortisol, and DHEA. We will talk about each of those in a bit of detail. The way these hormones are made is that first pregnenolone is formed, and then other hormones are made of it. It is a kind of master hormone producing the others from inside the adrenals. In addition, pregnenolone has been known for some time. We call all of these hormones "steroids" and that is kind of a funny term when you use it around people. People link steroids with steroid abuse in bodybuilders or they think about them as things like prednisone and steroid. Chemically, a steroid is any hormone that is built on cholesterol and that is all the hormones from the adrenals and the testicles and the ovary. They are all steroids by that definition so it is not a loaded term or anything inherently bad.

So pregnenolone is one that is known to have a big effect on the brain function as well and it is been shown to be powerful for affecting memory in animals and human beings, more than many other hormones or many other treatments. If someone is lacking it, it can substantially diminish short-term memory and longer-term recall. Adequate amounts of pregnenolone can reduce some negative effects from stressors. The levels of pregnenolone, like many hormones, generally do go down as we age so we expect to see lower levels over the years and in almost anyone. It is good to understand that it is should be screened or tested because the levels should be age-appropriate. However, people can commonly become lacking each decade they make it. A group of brain chemicals made as well from pregnenolone is called neurosteroids. They are a big part of helping the brain signal properly and help a good mood and memory and mental alertness as well. Overall lack of pregnenolone parallels much of the complete aging process.

It is been known about for some time. There were some studies done on human beings in the 40s and they were giving factory workers pregnenolone to see how it would affect their general fatigue and their functionality. It was also studied as a possible anti-inflammatory. Around this time though, there was also research going on with many other adrenal hormones and their synthetic analogs. So the research quickly moved towards more powerful, more quick-acting adrenal hormones like cortisol, then also synthetic analogs of it such as prednisone. In addition, they saw that these hormones in high doses had dramatic effects on stimulating activity and reducing inflammation. It took a little while longer to see how substantial the side effects could be from those compounds when given in high dosages. Consequently, much preliminary research on pregnenolone was done and was encouraging, but was dropped when everyone thought that cortisol was just the be-all-and-end-all and answer for almost all medical problems.

Pregnenolone can also get low when there is generalized stress on the adrenal glands. That comes about from what we call stress in day-to-day life. Our stressors – whether they are physical or psychological – they cause us to go into a fight-or-flight state and that state causes our body to make a little more energy than it would normally. Ideally, that state would not last for long. So commonly, we stay stuck in that fight-or-flight state for long periods. The fight-or-flight response is a mechanism that evolved when we had more stressors that are physical. We were literally fighting or running.

Our body would release adrenaline and that would cause us to go into this state where our heart would beat a little faster, our blood would move away from our digestive organs into our skeletal muscle and we could then run a little faster or fight a little harder. However, that state was not good for us. The expectation was that it would not last for long. The state could be turned off only by a hard, physical response. When we are put into that state, we would respond to it and we would literally fight or run. Once done, it was over, then the body turned off the fight-or-flight response, and mechanisms would occur afterward to heal the stress and the efforts from the high output of energy.

However, the big issue we face now in the modern world is that we have so many triggers that that we do not respond to physically – that are just not appropriate. You know we have relationship, financial, deadline stressors – you name it – and these are all things that we do not physically fight or physically run from. Consequently, they turn on the stress response just as if we were chased by a tiger but we do not engage these stressors physically. Consequently, we do not move out of the stress response. For many people whose lives are sedentary, that may go on all the time. Chronic stress is a big part of poor depth of sleep and poor quality of sleep, then that becomes a vicious circle. When we do not sleep well we do not get proper repair of our bodies and proper restoration of our immune function.

So chronic stressors can strain the glands and cause unhealthy amounts of hormone to be made. This can manifest in many ways. It can be just anger, edginess, fear, or anxiety from someone being overworked physically or mentally. We can also see this in someone overtraining – too much intense exercise, too many back-to-back workouts, not enough rest days. This can create stressors on pregnenolone and adrenal hormones as well. Temperature extremes – when it is hot or cold –can be a factor. Exposure to various types of toxins, rather common in the modern world, then being low in some important nutrients can do it as well – so big factors that many of us have some going on.

Symptoms that make us think about pregnenolone being low and adrenal dysfunction in general, would include feeling more weak than we would expect. Our temperature being low, having a difficult time growing muscle tissue properly, our blood sugar not being stable – having big blood sugar fluctuations, our memory not as good as it could, indigestion, easy confusion; being hungrier than we would expect can be factors as well. This list also includes not being able to concentrate well and higher allergic responses. Think about someone developing more and more allergies. In these cases, it is good to think about adrenal dysfunction as possible culprit behind that. Feeling frustrated and edgy, digestive changes – diarrhea and constipation, especially when they fluctuate back and forth. Other symptoms include feeling lightheaded or dizzy – this is prevalent if someone has that happen right when they stand up. For example, you are sitting or lying for a while and you get up quickly and feel dizzy or faint for a bit. There is a name for that. We call that orthostatic hypotension and that strongly does point primarily toward there being some stress on the adrenal glands.

Other symptoms include cravings for salty things, cravings for sweet things, and the skin being thinner or dry – which can also go with thyroid disease of course. Premenstrual symptoms, also airborne allergies can be more severe. Some with adrenal dysfunction do not sweat well. They will say, "Hey, I'm out in the heat. I'm being active" but they just do not sweat that readily and that can be part of this. In addition, low blood pressure can be a factor. Those who have abnormally low blood pressure – perhaps less than 90/60 on occasions –can be a sign of a weak adrenal function. We seem the same with palpitations – which can be from poorly regulated blood pressure – and we might see intolerance of alcohol where small amounts that can be consumed normally without effect could cause more intense disorientation or a more substantial hangover, and that can be a sign of there being weak adrenal glands.

Now another big hormone, in terms of the hormones the adrenal glands make, is DHEA. DHEA is more of an androgenic hormone, more of a male-like hormone. The androgenic hormones are involved with the growth of muscle tissue and some male characteristics such as body hair. This is also the principal source of testosterone in women's bodies. A little of this is made into testosterone in men's bodies – not as much. It is also a source of some estrogen so it goes both ways. As an androgen, it has roles to play in helping bone develop properly. If DHEA is lacking, that is one more factor making bones less strong or less healthy. It also affects growth of muscle mass – the spontaneous growth of muscle mass.

When DHEA is lacking or well below a healthy range, someone will tend to be heavier than they would be otherwise and have greater body fat – greater relative percent body fat – and less lean mass. This does also tend to have an effect on exercise capacity correspondingly. If you have less muscle, you will not train as well and you will not recover as effectively. DHEA is also a hormone that is involved with converting thyroid hormone – making T4 into the more active T3. Sometimes, if someone converts poorly and is low in DHEA, that is the only culprit and treating DHEA can be a benefit for that. Overall, it reverses the negative effects of cortisol so cortisol – or too much of it – wears the body, breaks it down, makes us lose our muscle and can make us gain fat more easily. DHEA is the counter for this.

In a perfect scenario, if we experience short-term stressors then we make high cortisol but we also make high DHEA to counter the negative effects of the cortisol and this is called the stage one stress response. What can happen if stressors go on for long, long periods, the cortisol may stay high – the body is still working hard to engage the stressor – but there is too little pregnenolone left to make DHEA out of. Pregnenolone makes both cortisol and DHEA, but in finite amounts. If stress goes on too long, pregnenolone starts to be diminished as more of it goes over to cortisol. However, your body has to keep going but less is available to form DHEA so there is less repair happening, and this is the stage two of the stress response. Then if it keeps going on for longer periods, eventually there is so little pregnenolone that both hormones start to diminish and we see low levels of DHEA and low levels of cortisol and that is the stage three stress response. That is kind of the hardest one.

Cortisol is a little different from the other two in one big way as it is circadian or diurnal, meaning that cortisol is not made in the same amount all day. A healthy person will make extremely different amounts of cortisol at various times of day. Ideally, what would happen is that the primary spike of cortisol is made right about when you wake. I think about this as the internal coffee machine and that is what is happening. When your body makes a big surge of cortisol that is what makes you not sleep and that is what makes you start to wake and want to get out of bed and start doing things. There is a morning spike that is normal and healthy, and you could guess that those who do not make this good morning spike do not wake as energized. As the day progresses, cortisol is made in smaller and smaller quantities and it diminishes. It starts to drop around noon and it should be dropping clearly by afternoon. Ideally, when we are going to sleep there are trivial, if any, amounts of cortisol being made as it shuts off. Cortisol is one of the principal factors regulating our sleeping and waking cycles.

Now you may have heard about melatonin. That is a nighttime hormone made by the pineal gland, a small thing inside the brain. In a healthy system, melatonin and cortisol are opposites. When you are making plenty of cortisol, you would not be making melatonin, and vice versa. If cortisol does have a good spike in the day, then a drop off later in the day stimulates the nighttime secretion of melatonin. If cortisol is not made in a high enough amounts early or if it is not dropping off rapidly as the day progresses, you do not get that surge of melatonin at night –a big part of not getting good-quality restorative sleep and that further disrupts the whole cycle. It further makes it more difficult to create cortisol at the right times. Cortisol is unique in that it is diurnal.

Now what its jobs are – it is a big factor for bringing proteins into the blood and the liver – amino acids specifically. That is important for regulating blood sugar and tissue growth. If the rate is incorrect, however, then we break down muscle mass – a considerable problem. It also helps the liver convert amino acids to glucose, part of how the liver makes energy. So if cortisol is not functioning right the liver does not have good amounts of its own energy source and that is a big part of why we can see people that have issues with detoxification not working as well because they have poor or abnormal cortisol output. It is also part of breaking down fats for energy. Now a paradox though is that if there is too much, the body cannot effectively break down fat tissue and we get more storage because cortisol does also make us more resistant to insulin over time if there is too much of it. It is also part of helping us manage our stress response to infections, changes in temperature, emotional traumas and it is a factor in our mood. When cortisol fluctuates, we feel just more stressed, literally. We feel more frantic and more upset and things affect us more strongly.

In general, when too much cortisol makes us less able to burn glucose inside our cells, that means we have to store more glucose leading to fat formation. Several years ago, there was an aggressively marketed product called CortiSlim. In the public's mind – that product linked cortisol as a hidden problem with obesity – and for some it is. Ironically, the product was a stimulant that was not regulated. If anything, stimulants raise cortisol – they would not lower it as it promised. Excess cortisol can be a factor in making us more likely to store sugar rather than burn sugar. It does also make us break down proteins. It can also make our bones thin. Too much of it can also hurt skin repair – make us not heal properly – and it can suppress the immune system, especially the system that protects us against things entering our bodies. We see this when we make too much cortisol, which happens even if we are taking cortisol as well. Cortisol in various forms is used as an agent to lower inflammation and there are many synthetic analogs of cortisol used for this purpose especially. Prednisone, medrol, and hydrocortisone are examples of this. They are effective at lowering symptoms quickly but they are high in side effects. They should be avoided or used cautiously and with the understanding that there can be major side effects.

So overall, a big, part of cortisol's job is regulating our blood sugar. The more erratically the food enters our bloodstream – the more we are erratic about the timing of our food – the more we have to make our adrenal glands work to keep our blood sugar in the right range. One of the easiest things we can do to make life easier for the adrenal glands is to eat regularly and keep our blood sugar well managed.

With the adrenals and the thyroid, part of the relationship in a little more detail is that cortisol is also a big part of how we make T4 into T3 outside the thyroid. So even if your thyroid is working perfectly the cortisol – if it is lacking – that will not convert the hormone into the active type so you will still feel like there is too little. On the other hand, if there is too much then that will block your cells from using the T3 after you make it. So it has to be dialed in to have things work properly. Now the adrenals, they do have more severe diseases too. They can just about shut off and we call that Addison's disease or severe adrenal insufficiency. It is a little less common but it does happen. Much more common is to have simple underperformance of the glands.

So how do we sort this? Well, like many things we want to measure the hormone output from the glands. The adrenals can be a little more involved, kind of like the thyroid. One factor is the issue of the broad normal range. The laboratories' normal range often does not distinguish time of day. Consequently, a level that would be normal at one time would not be another time. Another issue is that someone can have problems with cortisol some times of the day but not others. Therefore, if you are not checking at the right time you may not see that it is an issue.

There are tests that also measure cortisol in the urine and that can help get a sense of how much you make over the day as an average but usually when we are looking at more subtle problems of the adrenal glands, it is not as useful. There are tests that use saliva, which can reasonably accurately measure cortisol from a spit sample and the advantage of that is that allows us to collect many different samples across the course of a single day and that can show how the whole day's curve or cycle is working – how much you are making morning, noon, afternoon and nighttime. For some, the amount they make at one of those times could be just right on – fine – but for others that could be the one time where it is a problem. Therefore, it is good to screen the whole day, especially initially. This can be measured in blood as well. There can be a disruption of cortisol just by a blood draw. That can actually cause the scores to be altered somewhat. This is a problem with blood tests for cortisol.

Tests can also show how you make it in response to a challenge – meaning how you would make it if your body asked you to make more – and this is helpful if you think there is some degree of adrenal compromise as well. In this case, we give a low dose of what your body would use to help signal the glands, and then measure how much cortisol elevates afterward. It is called an adrenal challenge test. Probably the single useful thing though is the salivary studies for seeing how much is made and how the day's cycle fluctuates and from that, you know whether the problem is simple over-activity or under-activity of cortisol or if it is a variation.

The DHEA and pregnenolone – they can be measured rather easily through the blood or the saliva. The blood is not bad and it is actually good because it is generally not an out-of-pocket expense. In addition, blood tests work well because those hormones are stable throughout the day and not as diurnal. A single reading is more meaningful and can make more sense out of single time. Those hormones are actually rather easy to replace as well. If they are lacking to a small degree they can be used in oral forms. There are no typical side effects or complications with most low dosages. If someone does not need it, and they take an excessive dose or if they do not lack it at all then they can have side effects of excess. Both are similar. Both can create side effects that include jitteriness or anxiety or palpitations. This is especially true for DHEA. We can also see androgenic side effects like facial hair growth or acne or even thinning of head hair.

They are powerful hormones. It is a bit of quirk that they are non-prescription. There was a change in legislation a little more than thirteen years ago, which allowed that to happen and many were not pleased with that. However, they are powerful hormones and they can have complications and side effects if they are taken in wrong amounts. However, people with chronic inflammatory states such as arthritis especially, are often low in these hormones. They are one thing the body would make to stop inflammation and they may not be making it well enough. If they are brought back to a healthy range, they can give some benefits that would be obtained from stronger oral steroids like prednisone but with generally much higher safety profiles. They are useful.

Typically dosages for DHEA, suggest some men can need as little as five milligrams. Rarely would you need more than fifty, and the most common is between ten and twenty-five. With pregnenolone, roughly the same dosing is used but just doubled, so men would typically need between twenty-five and a hundred milligrams if they were extremely low. The smartest thing for any type of replacement regime is to start within the low end of the scale and retest and adjust as needed. Women need smaller dosages for both and commonly if they take too much, especially DHEA, they can get side effects such as the facial hair growth, the acne or the head hair thinning or the palpitations. If they are low, they may just need a few milligrams and that can be sufficient for them.

With Cortisol, the hormone can produce a simple deficiency or a simple excess or more commonly a disturbance in the day's rhythm.

When there is a simple deficiency, it is extremely rare that a cortisol replacement is needed. That is generally the case when we think about Addison's disease or more of a severe loss. It is something that one should not go into too casually. The difficulty is that because cortisol is so tightly controlled and made at such different amounts at various times of day if you do start taking it from outside your body you get less control about how you regulate it inside your body and that can be a considerable problem. Cortisol replacement therapy should not be started too lightly and it should be made clear that there can be issues, complications, and side effects. Long term, oral use of cortisol can thin the esophagus, thin the bones, and create problems of excess cortisol, even if only small amounts are needed.

Most commonly, we try to help the body use it more effectively. One of the easiest ways for this is using licorice. The neat thing about licorice is that it delays the rate at which your body eliminates cortisol so by using it, it can gently elevate the levels without giving you more cortisol as such. In many cases we are looking at not so much a simple deficiency but more so an imbalance of how it is made throughout the day. It could be too little early in the day and too much later in the day. That is getting more recognition in the medical world as a real problem to health and a real risk factor for total mortality. Therefore, it is good to be aware of it and it is good to correct.

There are some fats, which help the communication between the pituitary, the hypothalamus, and the adrenal glands, and these are mostly versions of phosphatidylserine, a fat that regulates how all of them communicate to bring cortisol back into a state of balance. It is primarily lowering so if it is being taken orally, the principal strategy is to take it during the times of day when you would want cortisol to reduce, which are primarily nighttime or close to bedtime. However, over time, it resets that rhythm making it remain stable and more normal, and this is a situation where many adaptogens can be used – many good plants like ashwaganda or rhodiola or some milder versions of ginsengs such as Siberian ginseng can help. Schizandra is also a useful plant – a useful substance for this – as is basil or Tulsi – the holy basil – and these adaptogens tend not to be disruptive but more so resetting. They can help correct the timing and the rhythm of the adrenals and all of them have some particular strength and merits but generally good tolerance and no big risks of toxicity or complications or side effects.

If we are seeing overall excesses of cortisol then it is more a matter of trying to regulate it with the intent of also suppressing it and a more useful strategy for this is Relora, a specific plant extract that has been well documented to diminish our cortisol response. There is a type of B5 called "pantothenate" that is also useful for this purpose – these are both safe with no big negatives. If cortisol is extremely high, other measures can be taken – there are cases where progesterone or oxytocin can diminish cortisol. The DHEA should be measured and should be regulated if cortisol is high because many negative effects are occurring also because of a possible lack of DHEA. Then finally, some antifungal medicines, such as ketoconazole, that tend to lower cortisol strongly, and sometimes side effect can be useful initially for resetting it when the glands are way off.

Chapter Summary

Adrenal activity varies greatly based on time of day. Stress and blood sugar are both managed by adrenal function. Many that feel tired or anxious after thyroid dose optimization have adrenal dysfunction. Conventional doctors only identify the worst forms of adrenal shutdown like Addison's disease and the worst forms of adrenal overactivity like Cushing's syndrome. Many with real adrenal issues make enough hormone but they make the wrong amounts at the wrong times. This is only detectable by salivary tests because they sample many readings over the course of the day.

Action Steps

26. Maintain regular habits of when you wake, sleep and eat. Think of your adrenal glands like babies, they do better on predictable schedules.

27. Brief intense exercise is good for the adrenals. Too little exercise, or prolonged low intensity exercise is not.

28. Eating foods that keep your blood sugar stable will also help your adrenal glands. These include lean proteins, vegetables, high fiber starches and healthy fats. Examples include poultry, mixed stir fry vegetables, pinto beans and almonds.

29. If lifestyle changes alone do not help, consider a combination of blood and salivary testing for adrenal function.

Chapter 10

Healing your Nervous System

Chapter At a Glance

- Role of the Nervous system and anxiety

- Fight or flight response

- Heart rate variability

- Sound light machines

- Yogic breathing

With thyroid disease, there can be a heightening of the body's stress response. In the short term, this can cause anxiety symptoms. In the long term stress reactions are self perpetuating. One of the key principles of our body's systems is adaptation. Anything we do a lot of we get better at. This is both good and bad. It is great when we exercise, bad when we get stressed. We have a voluntary nervous system and an involuntary nervous system. The voluntary system involves all the things we can control. I can consciously move my fingers to type these words, yet the rate at which my heart moves blood to my fingers is out of my conscious control. Some areas even have some overlap. My rate of breathing will be fine if I don't think about it, yet in a small act of defiance I can hold my breath or pant quickly.

Because the nervous system is so powerful, it can effect nearly any imaginable symptom. Some of the more common ones include fatigue, tremors, muscle cramps, numbness, tingling, twitching muscles, bloating, and joint pain.

Of course these can all happen for other reasons which is why this chapter is last. If you have done all the right things are still don't feel right, think about your nervous system.

The tough part is that conventional medicine really does not have any great treatment options for this. Sedatives can be given for acute states of panic, but they are neither safe nor effective for long term use.

The involuntary system has a gas pedal, the sympathetic nervous system and a parking brake, the parasympathetic nervous system. If we frequently go into a state of panic, whether by choice or not, it gets easier. This is especially true for stressors we go through early in life. These systems are switched back and forth via controls from 'group decisions' made by the hypothalamus, the pituitary and the adrenal glands. This group is referred to collectively so often, it is also known as the HPA axis.

A very measurable manifestation of HPA control is found in our heart rate. Of course our rate is effected by our level of cardiovascular health and recent activity. But even if we ignore how many times our heart beats per minute, we can constant changes in the duration between one beat and the next. For example, if we had a heart rate of 60 beats per minute, that would be an average of 1 beat per second. Yet if we carefully measure the duration between each beat, we would see that they are always above or below one second. We might go 1.1 seconds, 0.9 seconds, 1.2 seconds, 0.8 seconds and so on. Each time the heart rate speeds, the sympathetic nervous system is active, each time it slows, the parasympathetic is taking over for a fraction of a second. This interplay is known as cardiovascular entrainment.

For those who have endured excessive stressors for some duration, this ebb and flow does not go smoothly.

We all know that when we are frightened our heart speeds up but there is much more than that to it. Our heart is a dynamic participant in our mental state. There is a feedback loop between your Brain, your HPA axis and your heart. Any one of them can heighten or lower the stress response. You may have heard legends of yogis who could control their heartbeat at will. This is advanced but possible. A much easier and perhaps more practical feat is to be able to detect when our heart rate is out of coherence and to bring it back.

Entrainment can be easily quantified and, amazingly enough taken under conscious control. There are low cost devices consisting of nothing more than a wire with a finger clamp on one end and a usb port on the other. Basically you just plug it into your computer or PC and run the associated software while the sensor holds itself on your finger.

The display shows whether you are currently in coherence or not

By first seeing whether or not your heart rate is in entrainment or not, you become able to tell without using a device. The sensor comes with instructions and or software that walk you through basic mental techniques that restore a coherent heart rate.

It is like playing a video game, but the game is really the control of your involuntary nervous system. After a few sessions, the rhythm of your heart becomes quite obvious. After several more sessions, you get very good at moving it back to perfect coherence. These skills can then be applied to everyday life without the machine. You can be in the moment, feeling yourself getting stressed and consciously unwind the whole process before it gets to escalate and cause any problems. Like anything, the skill can diminish without regular use, but I've had many thyroid patients tell me that for years after getting the device and training with it they were able to control their stress response more easily than ever before.

Another way to improve brain function is to change the frequency of our brain waves. When we are chronically stressed, we get stuck in a state of highly rapid, inefficient brain waves.

Brain waves are electrical pulsations, like the heart rate but for the brain. It works by sending currents throughout the billions of nerve cells that make it up. How fast those signals get sent determines our state of awareness. These are quantified in HZ which equals the number of cycles per second.

Delta - 1 - 4 HZ - deep sleep

Theta - 4 - 7 HZ - creativity, spontaneity, emotional insight

Alpha - 8 - 12 HZ - relaxation, meditation, visualization

Beta - 12 - 20 HZ - analysis, mental focus

High Beta 20 - 40 HZ - fear, anxiety, chronic stress, nervousness

Normally throughout the day's cycle, we move from very slow delta waves when we are in deep sleep to faster beta waves when we are concentrating. Being in a state of chronic stress causes us to move into high beta waves which become a habit for our brain. This makes it harder to slow down all they way and be in states of relaxation or deep sleep.

This is something that we intuitively feel. So often people say things about how they can't sleep properly because their minds are racing. This is exactly what is going on. We spend too little time being physically active and too little time mentally relaxing. Also daily use of stimulants like caffeine can speed brain activity further. The paradox is that our brains don't work better when they are stimulated, they just get agitated and unfocused.

The leverage point is that our brains will mimic frequencies that our senses are exposed to. Light and sound work best, and they only work when they come in the range of frequencies our brain normally operates in.

Machines have been made that create pulses of light and beats of sound for the purpose of correcting our brain waves. Their cost has come down to a one time investment of as little as 100 - 150 dollars for machines that do a good job.

These are very helpful treatments for anxiety and insomnia. They really have a unique role because they are drug free, essentially free of side effects and in many cases their benefits persist well after usage stops. The one caution the manufacturers advise is for those prone to seizures from strobe lights.

Basically one would wear the device, especially at night time, to quickly wind down. They come with programs that start with pulses at higher rates, then quickly bring your brain waves down to desired states. Daytime programs are also made the encourage deeply refreshing alpha waves. In a matter of seconds, a user can experience the same benefits that would normally only come after years of meditation.

Alternate Nostril breathing

The yogis of ancient India were also aware that we had two opposing forces controlling us. These were portrayed as two serpents intertwining up our spine culminating at the nostrils. Of course, this image gave rise to the Greek Caduceus which we now recognize as the medical staff.

Like the Chinese the Yogis recognized specific channels though which our vital energies flowed. The Chinese called these meridians on which acupuncture treatment is based. The Yogis called these Nadis. The central two were the prime controllers of the others. Ida Nadi and Pingala Nadi (confirm which is which) sped and slowed the nervous system and were exactly like the modern concept of the sympathetic and parasympathetic nervous systems. The Yogis felt that these Nadis were fed through our breath. Specifically our breathing was said to shift in dominance from one nostril to the other in 90 minute cycles throughout the day. Modern research has shown that this does happen (confirm and reference).

Many patterns of disease and stress were ascribed to an

imbalance in the give and take between Ida and Pingala Nadi. One of the most effective and simple ways to correct this was by alternate nostril breathing. Modern research has confirmed that this simple technique has profound effects on chronic anxiety and stress.

To do the procedure, simply sit comfortably with the spine straight. Advanced modern Yogis/Yoginis are welcome to sit in full lotus. The rest of us can even do this well on a straight backed chair. The right thumb is used to block the right nostril by pressing the tissue above the opening against the septum. The right ring finger is used to block the left nostril.

The breathing pattern is to inhale on the left nostril while blocking the right, block both and hold the breath and then exhale out the right. Step two is to inhale right, block both and exhale left. Once one gets the basic technique down, the next step is to establish a rhythm.

The traditional method was to inhale on a 1 count, retain on a 4 count and exhale on a 2 count. If the room is quiet and you are relaxed, the best way to do this is by timing the breath to your heartbeat. In other circumstances, a second hand can work well. The flow is:

While blocking right nostril, inhale left nostril during 1 heartbeat,
Block both nostrils and hold for 4 heartbeats
Exhale out the right nostril for 2 heartbeats
Inhale right nostril for 1 heartbeat
Hold breath 4 heartbeats
Exhale left 2 heartbeats

This is one full round. As you do several rounds, it is normal for your breathing rate to slow dramatically. As this happens, double your count. Inhale on a 2 count, hold on an 8 count and exhale on a 4 count.

Five minutes daily can radically help anxiety and insomnia without side effects.

Chapter Summary

Your nervous system can cause many symptoms. The way your brain works, it is more likely to believe the symptoms are caused by anything other than itself. People with Hashimoto's disease are more likely than others to experience stress and anxiety. Like the rest of the body, the nervous system can heal.

Action Steps

30. Acknowledge that stress and anxiety can cause real physical symptoms

31. Create habits that allow your nervous system to relax

32. Unstructured journaling for a few minutes each day can be super therapeutic

33. Consider investing in mind body machines for high tech help

34. Learn and practice alternate nostril breathing for an easy solution you can use anytime

Closing

Thanks so much for spending some time with me. I am so excited to share this information with you because I have seen it help so many others in the past. Please value your health and act on this advice. Take each chapter and master it. Really understand the concepts and follow the action steps. Life can such a beautiful thing when you are healthy and inspired.

If you'd like to learn more or get more assistance, there are many great options. For personal coaching at a distance or to work with one of my doctors, learn more at www.integrativehealthcare.com. If you would like the audio program of this book visit http://www.myintegrativehealth.com. If you have not already read the Complete Idiot's Guide to Thyroid Disease, you can find it on Amazon, Barnes and Noble or at most bookstores.

I'd love to hear your feedback. Join me on Facebook at www.facebook.com/IntegrativeHealth.

In good health,

Dr. C

Alan Christianson, NMD

Acknowledgements

So many people have inspired my work in general and with thyroid disease specifically. My parents, Glen and Vivian come first. My mother read to me constantly as a child. This is how I learned to read so early and came to love learning. I'm blessed to have two sets of parents. My other father, David Frawley has inspired me about the power of the written word and the path of the author.

My wife Kirin and my kids Ryan, Celestina and Sawsan are my biggest sources of day to day joy.

Thanks to Miranda Helfrich, my operational manager and all the cool staff I get to hang out with at Integrative Health.

Huge thanks to Gena Lee Nolin, my 'thyroid sister' and her tireless crusade for the cause of Hashimoto's.

Special thanks to JJ Virgin and Brendon Burchard, for helping me dream big and always strive to do even more to help others.

About the Author

Alan Christianson is a Phoenix, Arizona-based Naturopathic Doctor (ND) who specializes in thyroid disorders. He founded Integrative Health, a group of physicians that focus on optimal wellness rather than disease. Accolades include Top Doc recipient in Phoenix magazine. Alan co-authored The Complete Idiot's Guide to Thyroid Disease. His numerous media appearances include The Today Show, CNN, The Doctors and Shape Magazine.

Made in the USA
San Bernardino, CA
24 November 2014